D1356930

THE HAIRY BIKERS'
ONE POT WONDERS

Si King & Dave Myers

THE HAIRY BIKERS'
ONE POT
WONDERS

CONTENTS

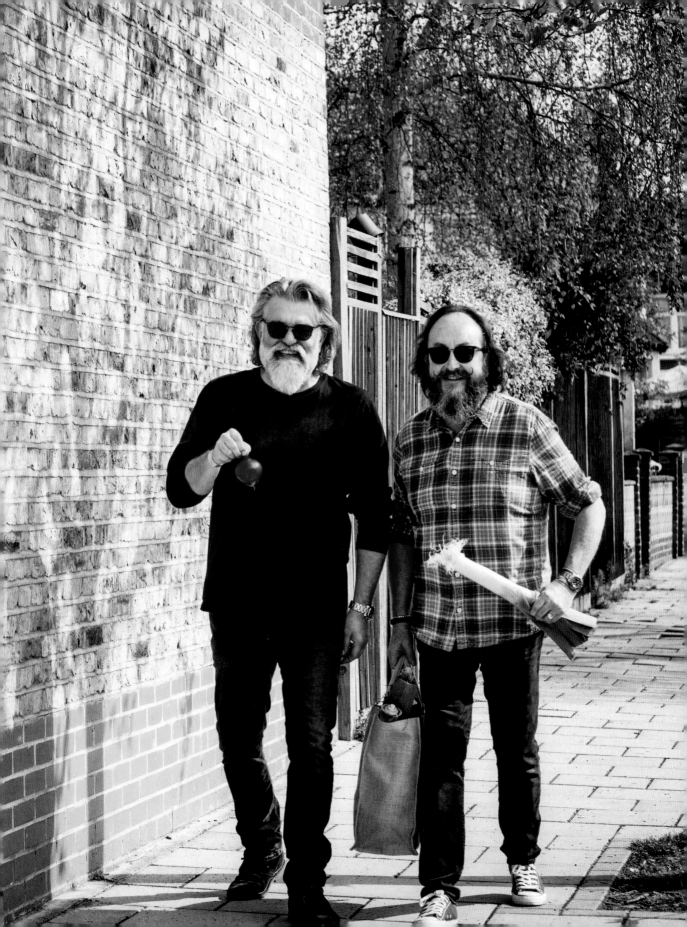

Great food, no fuss

As everyone knows, we love our food and we love cooking. There's nothing that pleases us more than putting something good to eat on the table, and we believe that the whole process of making a meal should be as enjoyable and fuss-free as possible.

That's why we decided that this latest collection of recipes should be our favourite one pots – food that you can prepare without using every bowl and pan in the kitchen. And not only are one pot meals time and labour saving – they also benefit from everything being cooked together, so all the glorious flavours are locked in and nothing is wasted. Just put the ingredients in the pan and let them work their magic. We're well aware that recipes like these are dishes that people really do cook. This is a book for everyday use – one pot cooking suits the way we live and the way most people live.

We've included plenty of classic one pots like soups and stews, but we've also come up with some cracking new ideas. Try our special one pot version of the full English breakfast, simple puff pastry tarts, tray bakes and pasta dishes – even mac 'n' cheese and a speedy spaghetti Bolognese. They're all meals you can cook in one pot, then take to the table so everyone can dig in and enjoy. And afterwards you don't have to face a sink full of washing up. The main meals all contain carbs, protein and veg so you don't have to add anything else, except a hunk of bread or a side salad if you feel like it. There are plenty of cakes and puddings too, and we've kept these sweet treats as easy to prepare as possible.

Some of these recipes are super-quick, so supper is ready before you know it. Others are simple to put together but then can be left to simmer and bubble away while you get on with something else – or put your feet up!

Whichever way, this is sharing food, food that will bring a smile to everyone's face – and won't leave the cook exhausted. We hope you enjoy making these recipes as much as we do.

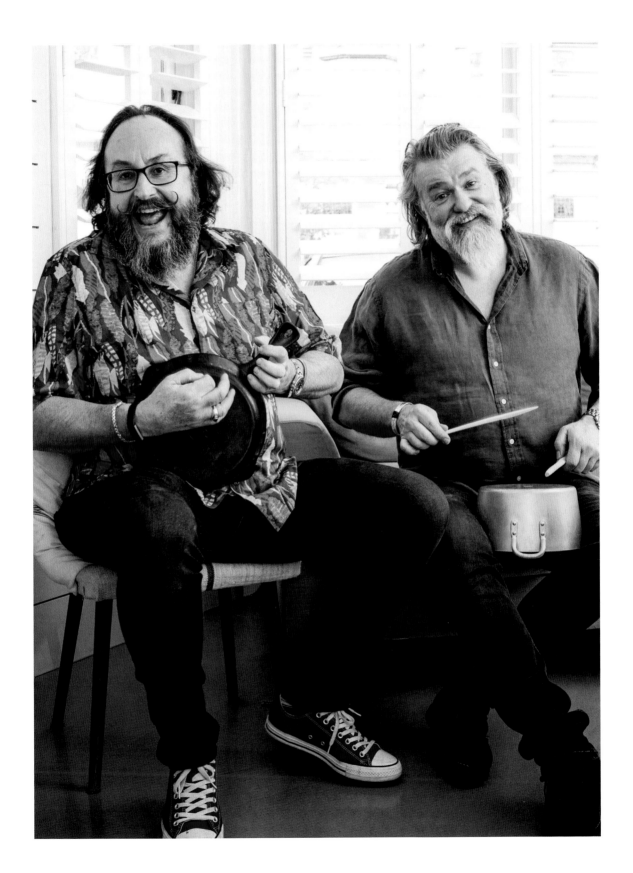

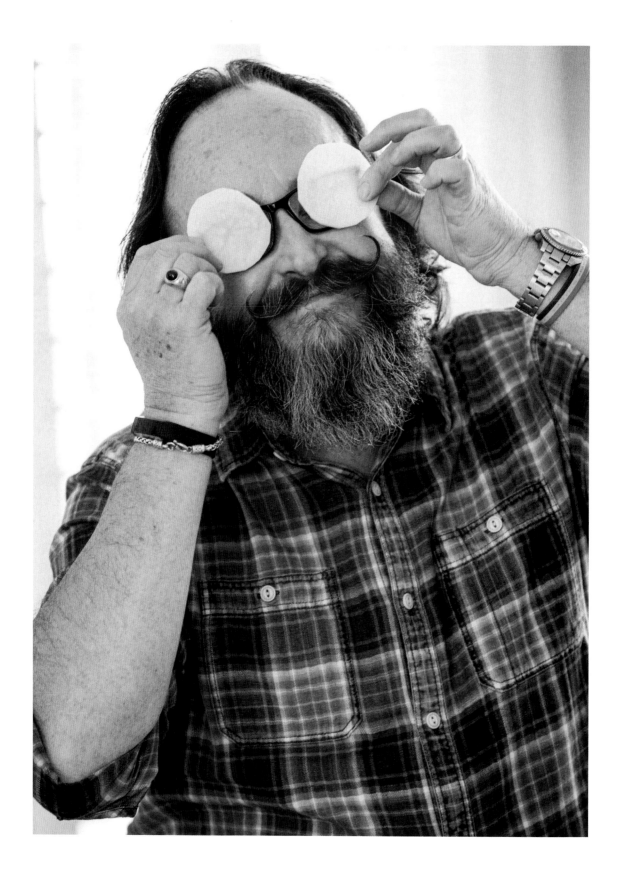

Dave:

The power of a one pot – I remember my mother's Lancashire hotpot, which was just so tasty. No flavours were wasted and we all used to love the crispy potatoes on top and the soft ones underneath, both cooked in the rich meaty juices. It's a simple assembly job, then the magic happens.

I love a tray bake, and as before, all the ingredients – protein, carbs, veg – work together to create something wonderful. And those little crusty bits that form round the edges of the dish are like culinary gold. There's huge pleasure in putting a one pot in the middle of the table and letting everyone help themselves. One of the things I like about one pots are that they are a democratic way of cooking – they're great for families and great for the busy lives that most of us lead, but they don't compromise on flavour.

These dishes all benefit from being cooked in one vessel, be it in a roasting tin, a casserole or a wok. You might need the odd bowl or two for some, but you won't end up with a kitchen sink full of washing up.

When I was a young lad, I used to cook flapjacks in a battered old toffee tray. Little did I know that those flapjacks and Mam's hotpot would be the inspiration for this book many years later.

_Si:_

Let's face it, everybody loves a one pot wonder. You can get really creative with the ingredients, then put them all together quickly and easily to produce a tasty lunch or supper for the household. I have very fond memories of my mam making one pot dishes for us when we were all at home. One particular meal that sticks in my mind was me mam's flat-rib broth. It filled the house with the homely smell of delicious cooking and the anticipation was sometimes unbearable because – as you won't be surprised to hear – we were always hungry in our house.

One pots are time efficient and the results, in our view, are always great, plus there's less washing up – what's not to love? For this book, we've come up with some excellent tasty recipes that we hope you will enjoy cooking for yourself and those you love.

So crack on and get stuck into the book. We've had an absolute ball putting all this together and the team has had a great time testing, tasting and reviewing the results. There have been a lot of one pots cooked in mine and Dave's homes. We really do hope you enjoy them all.

Notes from us

Peel onions, garlic and other veg and fruit unless otherwise specified.

Use free-range eggs whenever possible. And we generally use large eggs in our recipes unless otherwise specified.

Weigh all your ingredients and use proper measuring spoons. We've made the oven temperatures as accurate as possible, but all ovens are different so keep an eye on your dish and be prepared to cook it for a longer or shorter time if necessary.

We've included a few stock recipes at the back of the book and homemade stock is great to have in your freezer. But if you don't have time, there are good fresh stocks available in the supermarkets or you can use the little stock pots or cubes.

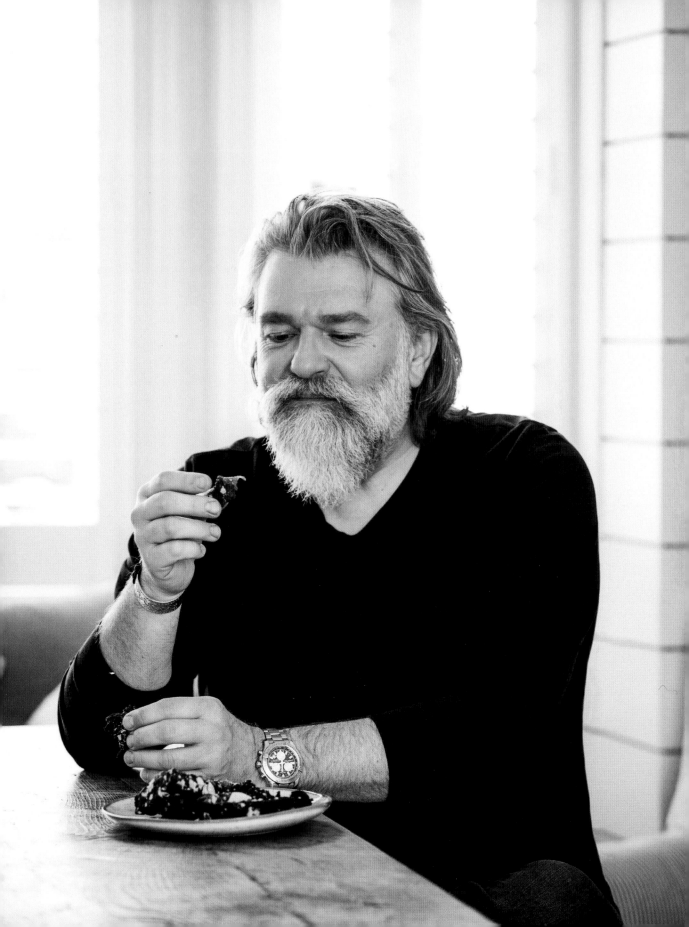

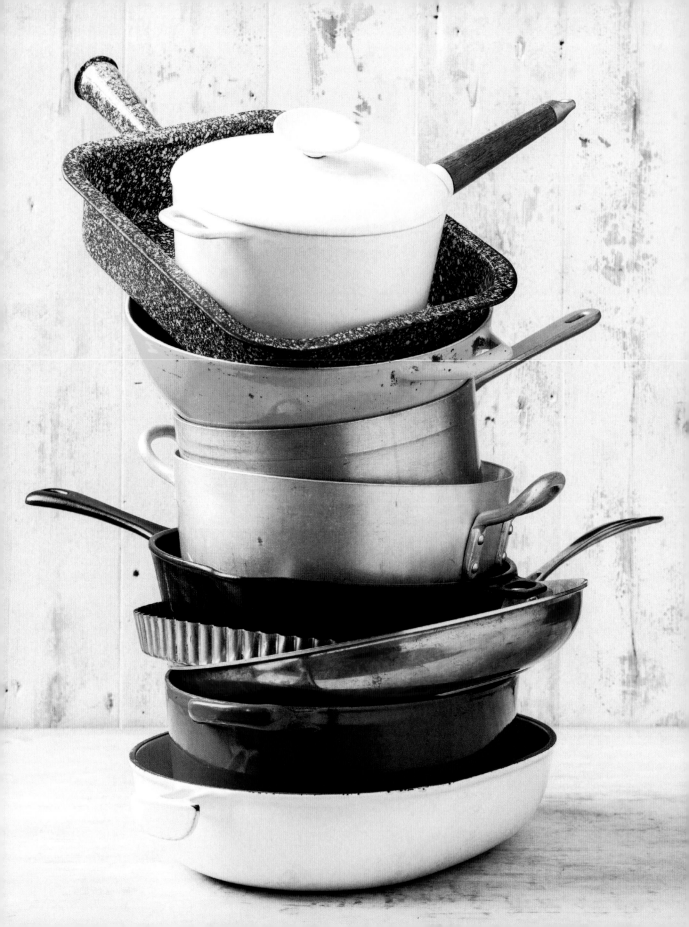

Pots and pans

We're not suggesting you have to buy every kind of pot and pan shown in this book but there are some that you will find particularly useful, if you don't have them already.

A flameproof casserole dish with a lid is perfect for lots of these one pot recipes. It's a great thing to have in your kitchen and a good one will last you for years. The enamelled cast-iron type is the best, as you can use it on the hob for browning meat and vegetables and then pop it into the oven to finish cooking the dish.

Obviously you need a couple of good saucepans, including a nice big one for soups and all-in-one pasta dishes. Heavy-based pans are best so you can leave them on the heat with less risk of the food sticking and burning. You'll need a non-stick or cast-iron frying pan too – we like the cast-iron ones, as you can put them under the grill and into the oven if you need to with no problems. A sauté pan, usually straight-sided and deeper than a frying pan, is also useful and it's good to have one with a lid.

Get yourself a sturdy roasting tin that you can use on the hob as well as in the oven. A baking dish that you can take to the table is perfect for tray bakes and crumbles. For the puddings and cakes, you might also want a brownie tin, a loaf tin and a good old-fashioned pudding basin.

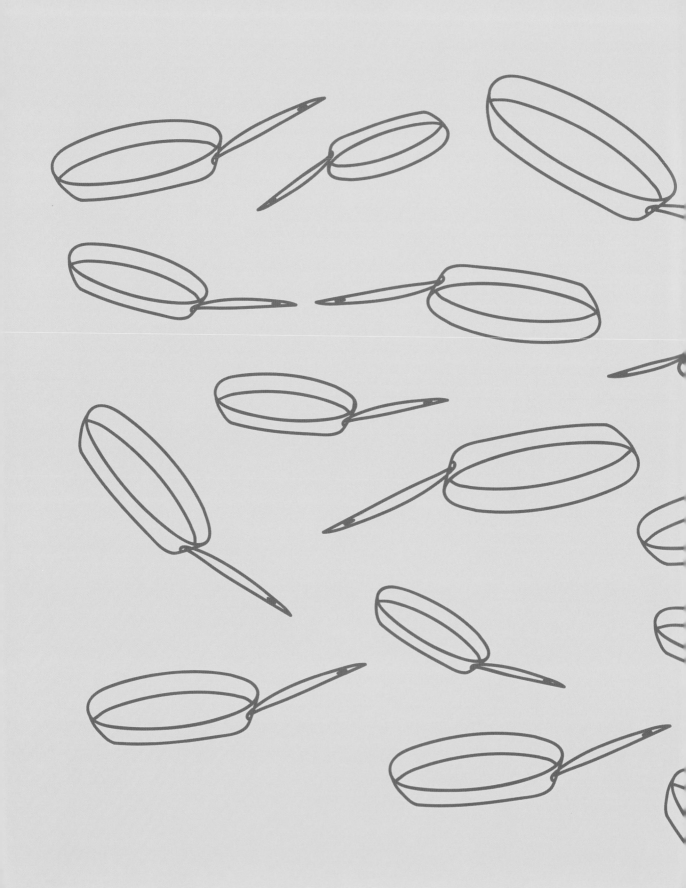

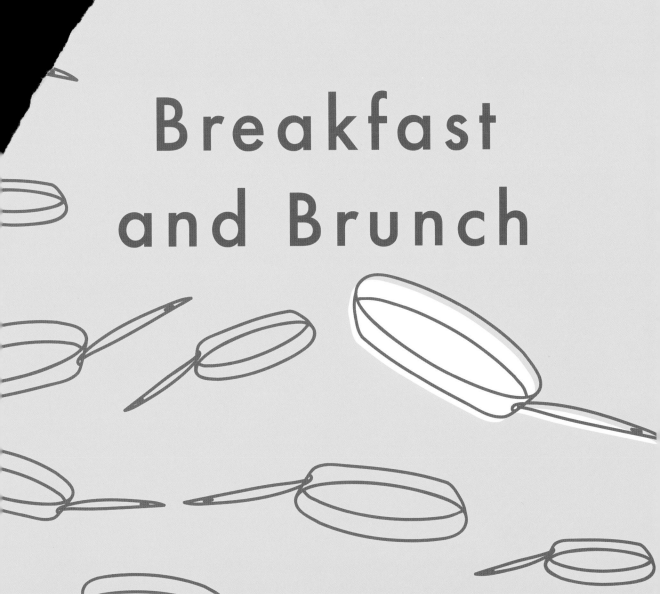

Breakfast
and Brunch

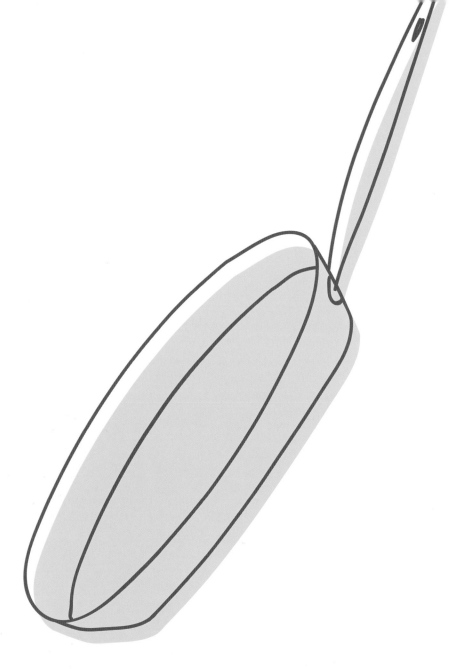

Our fruit and nut granola 18

Biker bircher 20

Full English shakshuka 22

Baked eggs with feta and tomatoes 24

Kedgeree frittata 26

Chorizo and prawn frittata 28

Savoury eggy bread 30

Banana French toast 32

Savoury Dutch Pancake 34

Raspberry, orange and honey muffins 36

Our fruit and nut granola

It really is worth making your own granola. It's a whole lot cheaper than shop-bought and you can put what you like into the mix – and control the sweetness. That's important because some granolas are loaded with sugar, and when we did our first Hairy Dieters book, we discovered that some so-called healthy granolas were more calorific than a fry-up! We like the dried mango in this recipe, but you can try papaya, pineapple and/or banana chips – whatever takes your fancy. Have a bowlful of this with some milk and perhaps some fresh fruit and you'll be well set up for the day.

Makes about 500g

250g porridge oats

50g desiccated coconut

150g cashew nuts, roughly chopped

pinch of salt

3 tbsp vegetable oil or melted coconut oil

50ml maple syrup

2 tbsp chopped stem ginger

1 egg white, lightly whisked

100g raisins

100g dried mango, chopped

Preheat the oven to 150°C/Fan 130°C/Gas 2. Line a large baking tray with greaseproof paper.

Put the oats, coconut and cashew nuts in a bowl and add the salt. Whisk the oil, maple syrup and stem ginger together, then pour them over the dry ingredients. Mix thoroughly. Pour the egg white over the oat mixture and mix again.

Spread the granola over the baking tray in an even layer, then press with the tips of your fingers at regular intervals to create small pockets – this will create more surface area and help the granola crisp up. Bake the granola for 50 minutes to an hour, but start checking after about 45 minutes. It's ready when it's golden-brown and crisp, but if the mixture feels at all damp, bake it for longer. When the granola is done, remove it from the oven and leave it to cool in the tray.

Transfer the granola to an airtight container and mix in the raisins and dried mango. It will keep for several weeks.

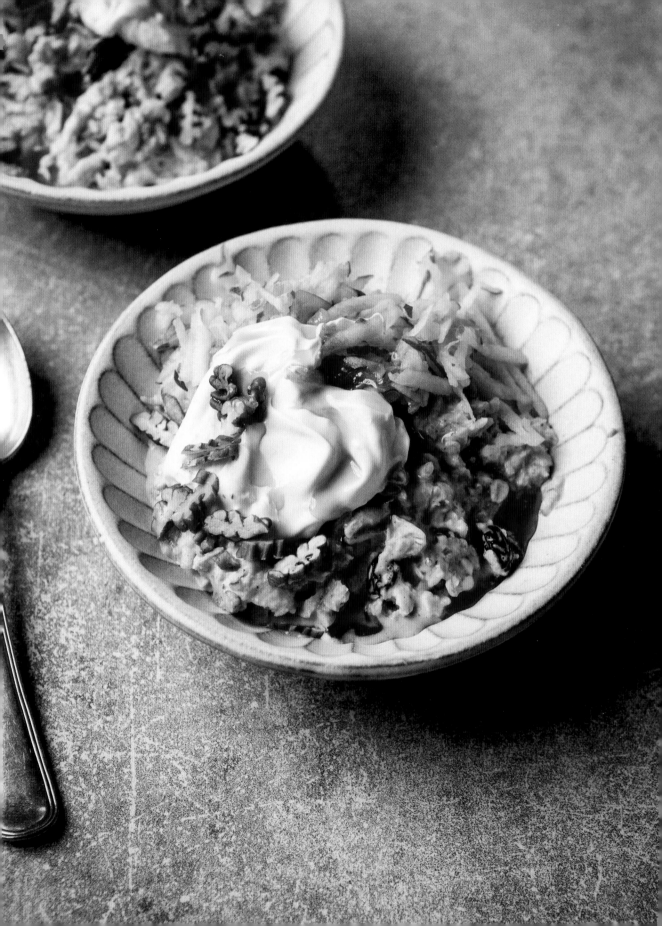

Full English shakshuka

We've taken the classic Middle Eastern shakshuka – one of our favourite dishes that we first discovered and cooked in Israel – and given it a touch of the full English to make an epic one pot breakfast or brunch. We've gone the full Monty here, but feel free to adapt as you like. A word of advice – this is proper filling, so you won't need lunch.

Serves 4

2 tbsp olive oil

6 sausages, peeled and broken up into balls

2 tbsp HP sauce

100g smoked bacon lardons

1 onion, thinly sliced

200g button mushrooms, halved

2 slices of black pudding (optional)

400g can of chopped tomatoes

100g haricot beans (about half a 400g can), drained and rinsed

4 eggs

salt and black pepper

To serve
hot buttered toast

Heat a tablespoon of the oil in a large frying pan or sauté pan that has a lid. Fry the sausage balls until they have browned on all sides, then add a tablespoon of the HP sauce. Stir to coat the sausage balls and keep stirring until they look caramelised, then remove them from the pan and set aside. Deglaze the pan with a little water and pour this over the sausages.

Add the remaining oil to the pan. Fry the bacon, onion and mushrooms together until the bacon has rendered its fat and is crisping up. The onion should have started to soften and brown around the edges. If using black pudding, crumble it up and fry it very briefly. Put the sausages back in the pan with everything else.

Add the tomatoes and the remaining HP sauce, together with the beans and about 200ml of water, then stir to deglaze the base of the pan. Season with salt and pepper, bring to the boil, then turn down the heat and cover the pan. Cook for 10 minutes.

Make wells in the mixture and break the eggs into them. Cover the pan and cook for a few minutes until the whites are just set and the egg yolks are runny. Serve with hot buttered toast.

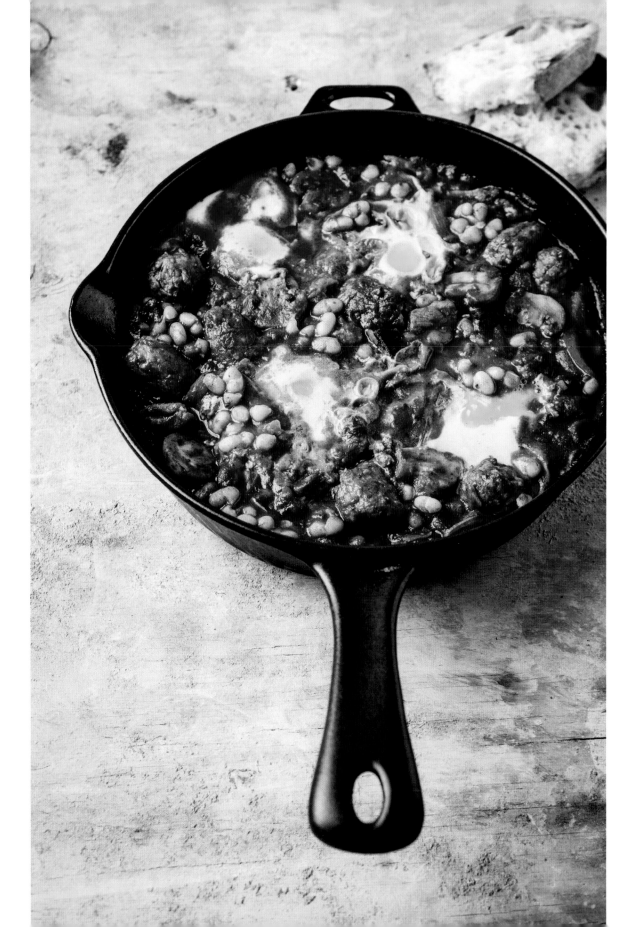

Baked eggs with feta and tomatoes

We think this makes a great family brunch or breakfast but it's good for supper as well. You can bake it in individual ramekins if you like but we prefer our one pot version. Serve with crusty bread.

Serves 4

2 tbsp olive oil

1 garlic clove, halved

8 tomatoes

1 small red onion, very finely sliced

a few fresh oregano leaves or ½ tsp dried oregano

8 eggs

200g feta cheese, crumbled

salt and black pepper

Preheat the oven to 180°C/Fan 160°C/Gas 4.

Brush the inside of a baking dish with the olive oil, then rub the cut garlic clove over it. Slice the tomatoes thinly, then gently push out the seeds. Put the tomatoes and onion in a colander and sprinkle them with salt. Leave them to stand for 15–20 minutes, then arrange them over the base of the baking dish. Season with plenty of salt and pepper, then sprinkle over the oregano.

Crack the eggs one at a time into a ramekin and pour each one over the tomatoes until they are almost completely covered. Sprinkle over the feta, concentrating it over the egg yolks – this will give them some protection from the heat, so they will cook less quickly than the whites.

Bake in the oven for about 15 minutes until the whites have set and the yolks are still runny. Serve immediately.

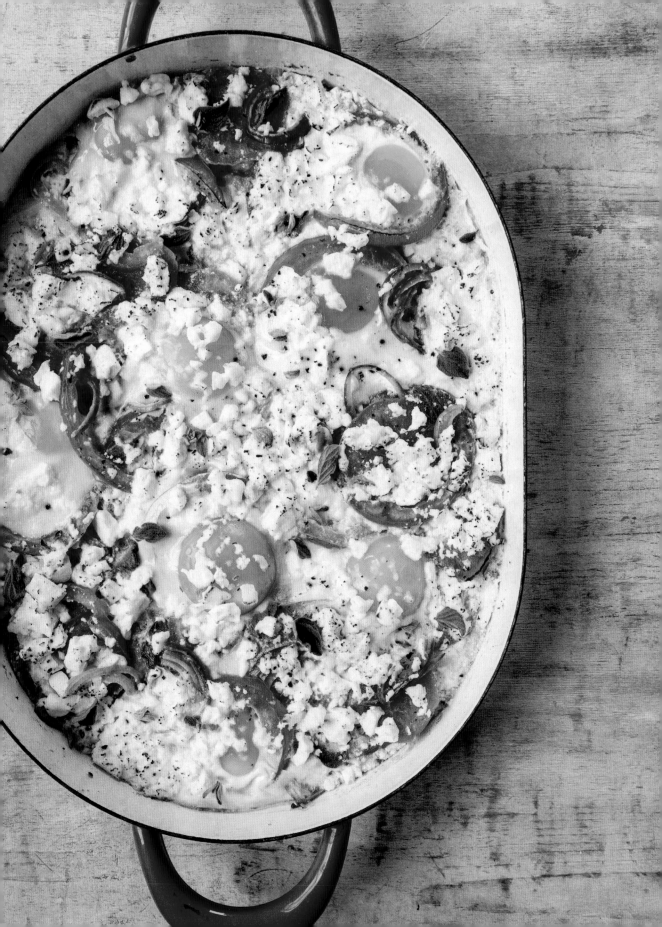

Kedgeree frittata

Once again, we've taken two of our old favourites and given them a new look – proper Hairy Biker fusion. Smoked fish goes so well with eggs that we thought it was just the thing for a frittata, and with the mild curry spicing it goes down a treat. Add rice if you have some around but this is fine without. Shop-bought mild curry powder is fine or try making your own with our special recipe on page 266.

Serves 4

1 tbsp olive oil

15g butter

1 onion, finely chopped

1 garlic clove, finely chopped

10g fresh root ginger, grated

1 tbsp mild curry powder

150g cooked rice (optional)

100g frozen peas, defrosted

6 eggs, lightly beaten

200g hot smoked trout or
   salmon

bunch of coriander, finely
   chopped

Heat the oil and butter in a large non-stick or cast-iron frying pan. When the butter has melted, add the onion and cook until it is soft and translucent. Add the garlic, ginger and curry powder and cook for a further minute, then add the rice, if using, and the peas. Stir to coat the rice and peas with the spices.

Pour the eggs into the pan and cook for a few minutes until the underside has set. Break up the trout or salmon into pieces and space these evenly over the frittata, then sprinkle with coriander. Leave the frittata to cook to a wobble or put it under a hot grill for a minute or so to finish setting it.

Leave to cool slightly, then cut into wedges to serve.

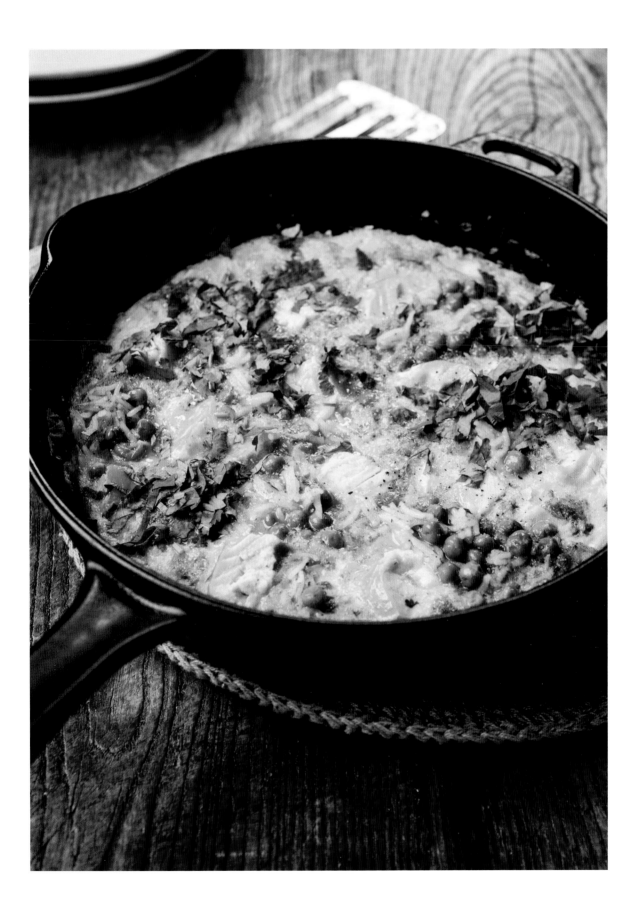

Chorizo and prawn frittata

We've got a bit of a surf and turf vibe going on here, which we enjoy. Chorizo is one of our favourite things and it goes so brilliantly with prawns. Try this – you're going to love it.

Serves 4

1 tbsp olive oil

150g raw peeled prawns

150g cooking chorizo, sliced

6 spring onions, green and white parts separated and sliced into rounds

6 eggs, lightly broken up (not whisked)

a few tarragon leaves, finely chopped

100g rocket leaves

salt and black pepper

Set a large non-stick or cast-iron frying pan over a high heat and add the oil. Add the prawns and cook them for a minute on each side until just pink, then remove them from the pan and set aside.

Add the chorizo and the white parts of the spring onions to the pan and cook until the chorizo has browned on both sides; the spring onions will cook very quickly in this time.

Spoon off some of the chorizo oil if it looks like there's too much. Season the eggs with salt and pepper and stir in the tarragon. Pour the egg mixture over the chorizo and cook for 2–3 minutes. Sprinkle over the prawns and the green parts of the spring onion. Leave the frittata to cook to a wobble or put it under a hot grill for a minute or so to finish setting it.

Remove the pan from the heat and sprinkle the rocket leaves over the frittata. They will wilt down slightly in the heat. Leave to cool for a few minutes before serving.

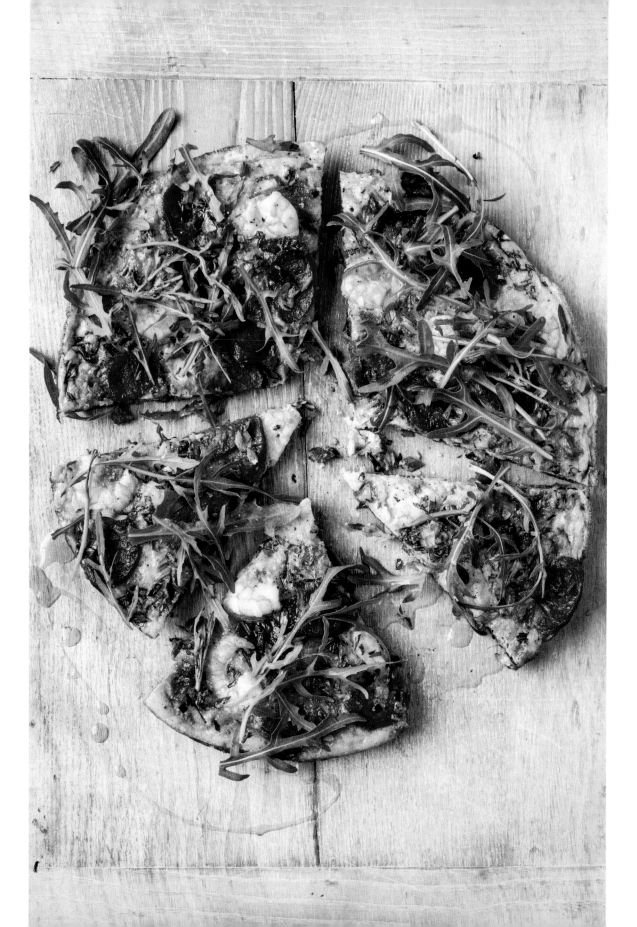

Savoury eggy bread

Oh my, this is eggy bread – or French toast – taken to another level, with a filling of cheese, mustard and a dash of good old tomato ketchup. We like putting the ham on top so it melts gently into the hot sandwich but you can put it inside if you prefer.

Serves 4

8 slices of granary bread

Dijon mustard, for spreading

4 thick slices of Gruyère cheese

tomato ketchup, for spreading

4 eggs

50ml whole milk

1 tbsp olive oil

knob of butter

8 slices of Parma ham

salt and black pepper

Spread 4 of the slices of bread with mustard and top with the slices of Gruyère. Spread the other slices with ketchup and make 4 sandwiches.

Whisk the eggs in a large, shallow bowl with the milk. Season generously with salt and pepper. Dip each sandwich in the egg mixture, making sure it is well coated by submerging it on both sides, then scrape off any excess egg that's clinging to it.

Put the oil and butter in a large non-stick frying pan. When the butter has melted and is foaming, fry the sandwiches until crisp and well browned on each side. Cut them in half and drape over the slices of ham, then serve at once.

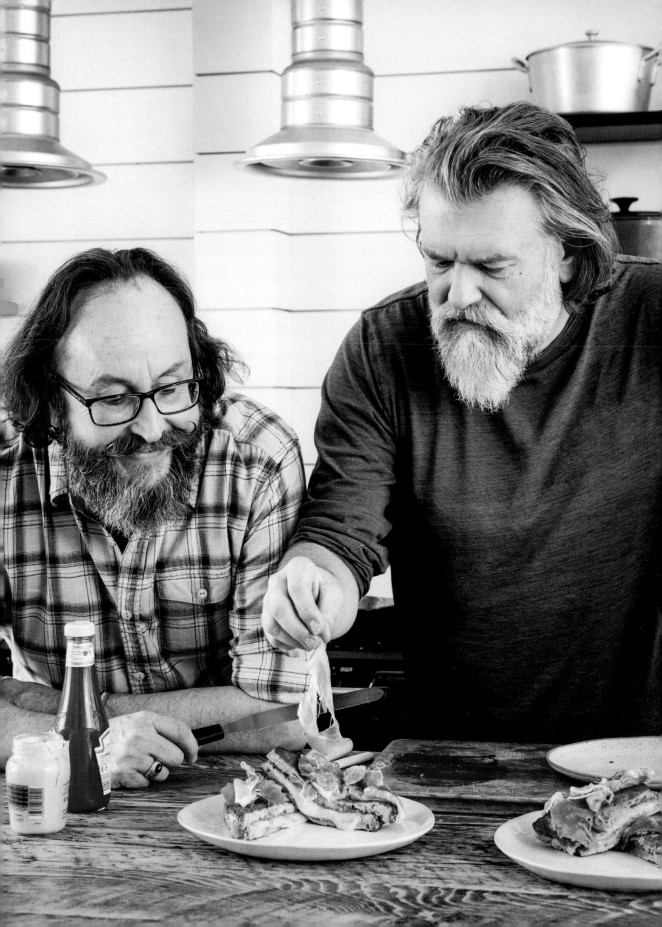

Banana French toast

Not one for every day but this makes a great treat for a cold rainy Sunday morning when you feel like some cracking comfort food. Brioche, bananas, peanut butter, cream – this is a big cuddle of a brunch and the sort of thing we think Elvis would have approved of!

Serves 4

8 slices of brioche

peanut butter and/or chocolate spread

2 bananas, sliced

3 eggs

2 tbsp double cream

1 tbsp maple syrup

½ tsp mixed spice

½ tsp vanilla extract

large knob of butter

To serve
demerara sugar

double cream or yoghurt

Lay the slices of brioche out in pairs. Spread them with peanut butter or chocolate spread – or use both if you like, one side of each. Arrange the banana over half the slices of brioche, then press the slices together to make 4 sandwiches.

Crack the eggs into a bowl and add the cream, maple syrup, mixed spice and vanilla extract. Mix thoroughly. Melt the butter in a large non-stick frying pan.

Dip each sandwich into the egg mixture, making sure it is well coated by submerging it on both sides, then scrape off any excess egg that's clinging to it. Fry the sandwiches in the butter for a minute or so on each side, until well browned and crisp.

Eat at once with a sprinkle of demerara sugar and some double cream – or yoghurt if you want to be a bit healthier.

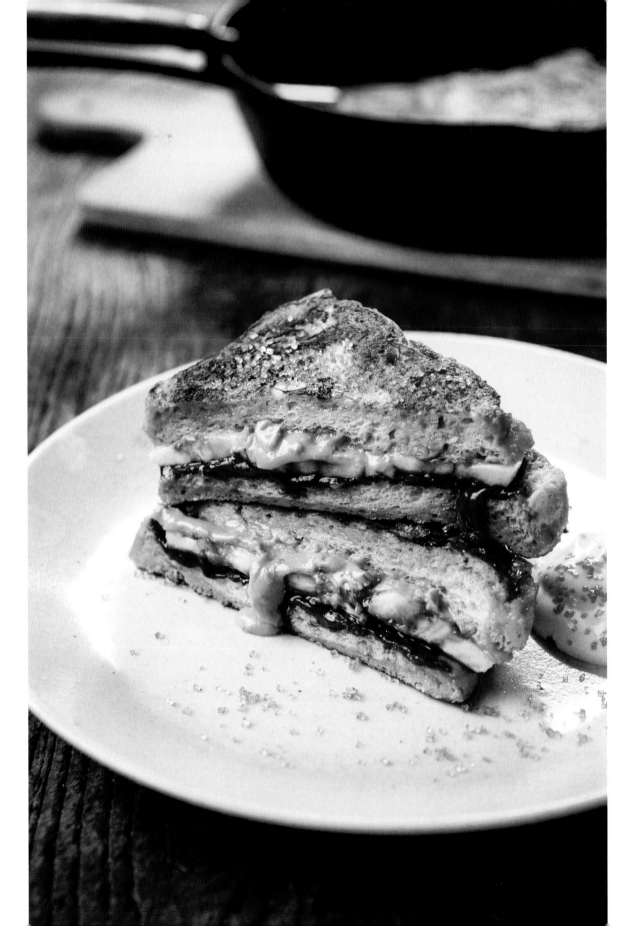

Savoury Dutch pancake

A true cross-cultural fertilisation that will make you smile – Yorkshire pudding meets a savoury bacon and Dutch cheese filling. The result is a scrumptious savouriness, which floats our boat as a brunch. This is quick to prepare and even quicker to eat.

Serves 4

Batter
75g plain flour
1 tsp rubbed sage
 (optional)
pinch of salt
3 eggs
125ml whole milk

Filling
2 tbsp vegetable oil or lard
75g smoked bacon lardons
2 shallots, finely chopped
1 eating apple, peeled and
 diced
100g Gouda cheese,
 grated
sage leaves, to garnish
 (optional)

Preheat the oven to 200°C/Fan 180°C/Gas 6.

First make the batter. Put the flour into a bowl with the sage, if using, and a generous pinch of salt. Work in the eggs to make a thick batter, then gradually add the milk until the batter is smooth and the consistency of single cream. Set it aside to rest.

Heat a tablespoon of the vegetable oil or lard in a large ovenproof frying pan or a roasting tin. Fry the bacon and shallots until the bacon is crisp and the shallots are lightly browned, then add the diced apple and cook for another couple of minutes. Remove everything from the pan and wipe over the base with kitchen paper.

Heat the remaining oil or lard in the pan or tin. When it is smoking hot, pour in the batter, swirling it round so the entire base is covered. Mix the cheese into the bacon mixture and sprinkle this on top of the batter, making sure you leave a wide border for the pancake to rise around the filling.

Put the pan in the oven and bake the pancake for 20–25 minutes, until it's lightly browned and has puffed up around the filling. Garnish with sage leaves and serve at once.

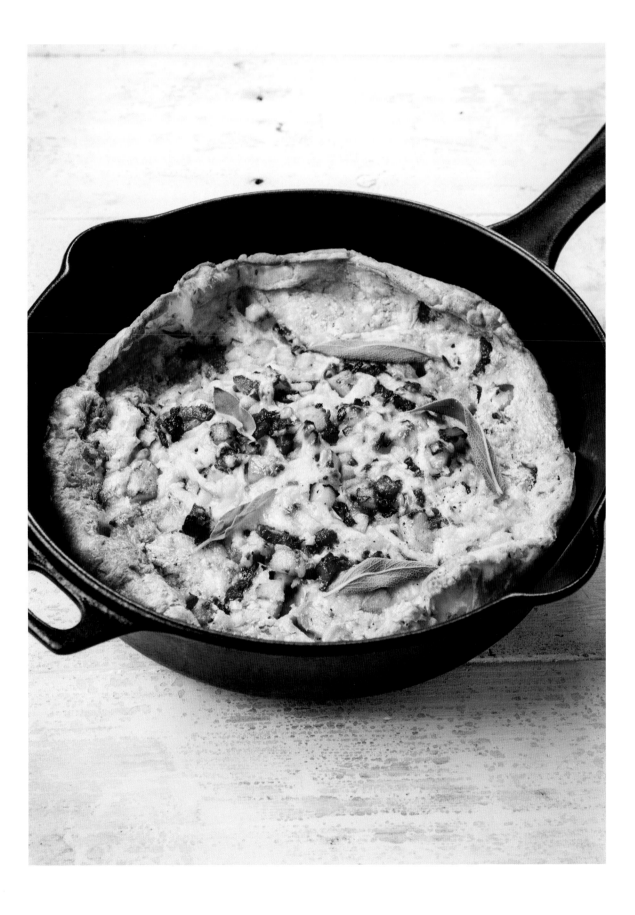

Raspberry, orange and honey muffins

Sometimes it's nice to have something sweet in the morning and we're big fans of a fruity muffin. What's more, these are muffins with attitude, containing oats and wholemeal flour so they're rich in fibre – that way we can have a couple without feeling too guilty! BTW, if you don't have any buttermilk you can make your own. Just add a tablespoon of lemon juice to 200ml of milk, stir and leave for 10 minutes.

Makes 12

200g wholemeal flour
50g porridge oats
2 tsp baking powder
½ tsp bicarbonate of soda
75g light soft brown sugar
pinch of salt
200ml buttermilk
75ml vegetable oil
25ml runny honey
1 egg
zest of 1 orange
150g raspberries

To serve
drizzle of honey (optional)

Preheat the oven to 180°C/Fan 160°C/Gas 4. Line a 12-hole muffin tray with paper cases.

Mix the flour, oats, baking powder, bicarb and sugar together with a pinch of salt. Whisk together the buttermilk, oil, honey, egg and orange zest. Combine the wet and dry ingredients, keeping the stirring to a minimum – it doesn't matter if the mixture looks lumpy.

Fold in the raspberries, again keeping stirring to a minimum, then divide the mixture between the muffin cases. Bake the muffins in the oven for 18–20 minutes, until they are well risen and springy to touch. Brush with the honey, if using.

Leave the muffins to cool in the tray, then transfer them to an airtight tin – if you haven't eaten them all!

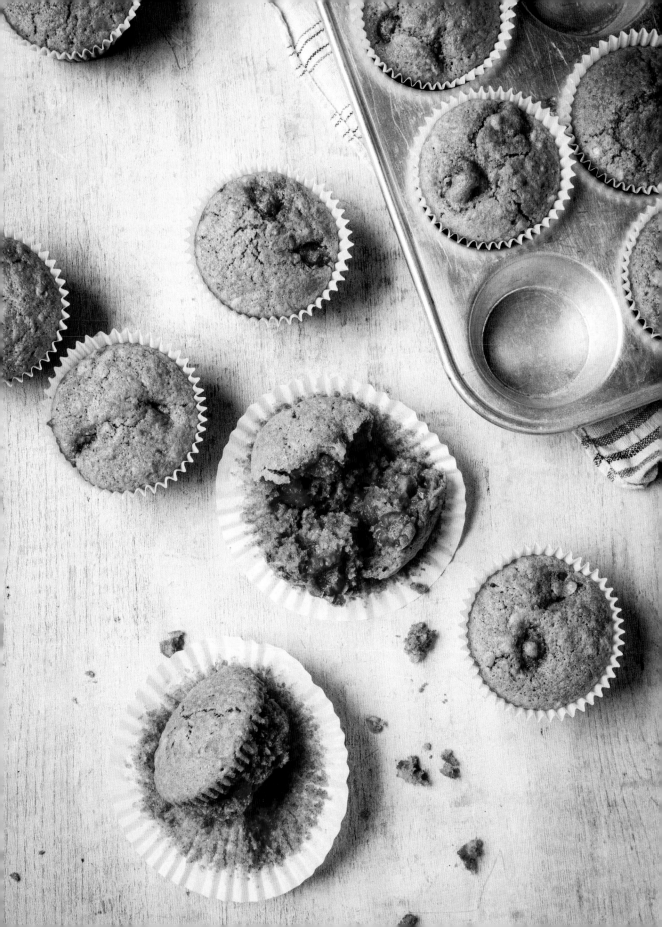

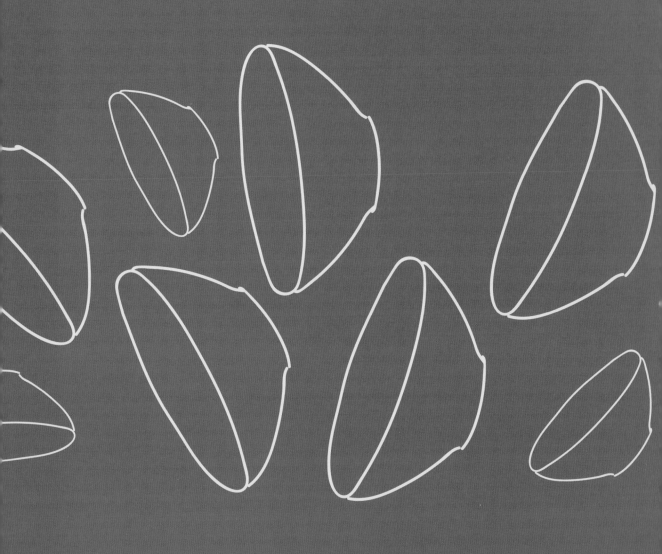

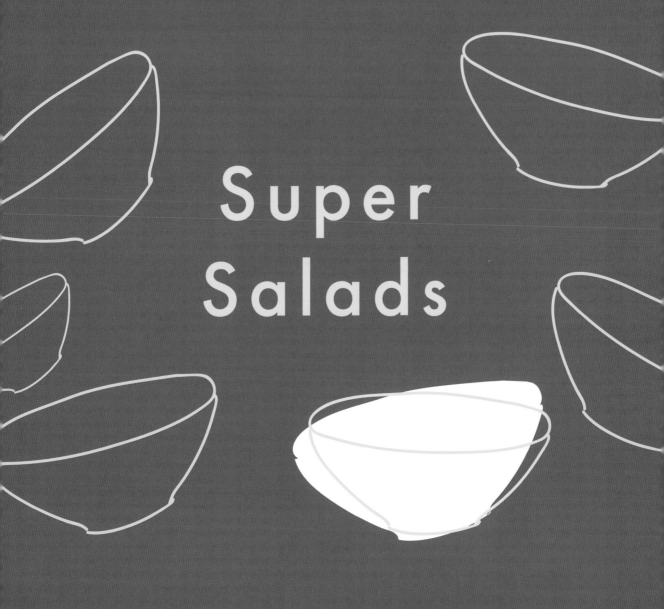

Super
Salads

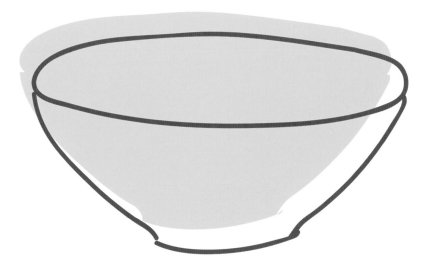

Chorizo and courgette salad 42

Cauliflower and lentil salad 44

Hearty ham and cheese coleslaw 46

Our big Biker tabbouleh 48

Succotash salad 49

Prawn, avocado and quinoa salad 50

Spicy couscous salad 52

Panzanella 54

Chopped chicken salad 56

Chorizo and courgette salad

The chorizo gives bags of flavour to this salad so you don't need garlic and lots of other seasoning. There's a lovely mix of textures too – a great meal in a bowl.

Serves 4

1 tbsp olive oil

100g cooking chorizo, diced

1 large red onion, finely sliced

2 courgettes, diced

400g can of cannellini beans, drained and rinsed

300g cherry tomatoes, halved

50g olives (black or green), halved and pitted

25g capers, drained

bag of baby salad leaves

a squeeze of lemon juice (optional)

salt and black pepper

Heat the oil in a large frying pan or sauté pan and add the chorizo. Fry it quickly until it's browned all over, watching it constantly – chorizo can cook very quickly and you want it to be well browned with plenty of fat rendered out, not blackened. Remove the chorizo from the pan with a slotted spoon and set aside. You need about 2 tablespoons of oil left in the pan, so spoon off any excess.

Add the onion and courgettes to the pan. Cook over a medium heat, turning regularly, until the onion has softened a little and the courgettes have browned – they should still be al dente.

Remove the pan from the heat. Put the chorizo back in the pan and add the beans. Stir so that everything is coated in the oil in the pan and season with salt and pepper. Leave to cool for a few minutes, so everything is just on the warm side of room temperature, then add the tomatoes, olives, capers and salad leaves. Toss everything together. Taste and add a squeeze of lemon if you like. Serve immediately.

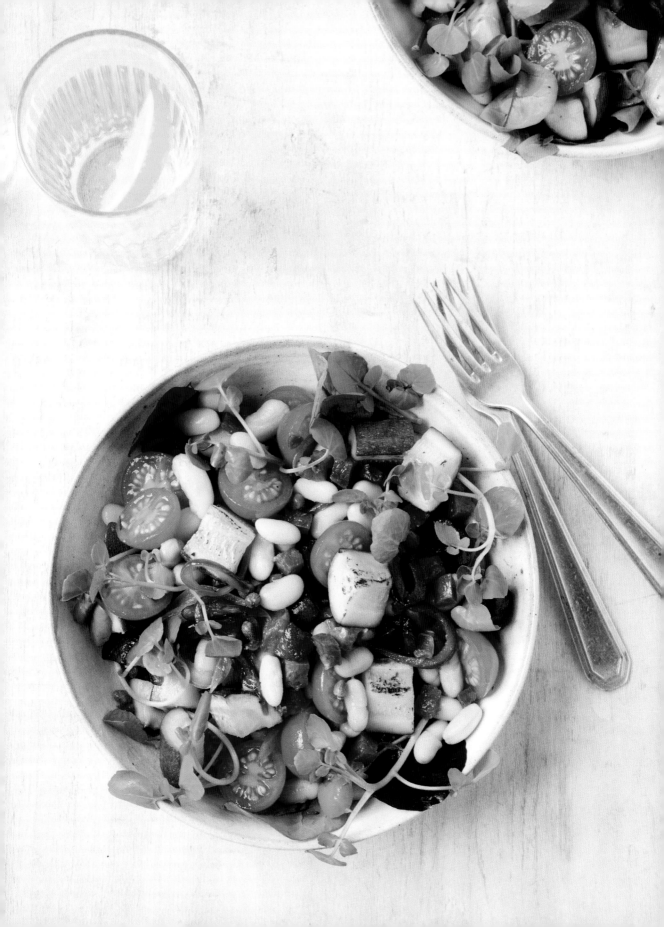

Cauliflower and lentil salad

We both love cauliflower and think that roasting really brings out its flavour. Cauli also goes beautifully with a touch of curry powder and this is a great salad for curry lovers! Adding lentils and green veg makes it both hearty and fresh – an ideal lunch with an Indian flavour.

Serves 4

2 tbsp flaked almonds

2 tbsp olive oil

1 medium cauliflower, broken into small florets

2 tsp curry powder

2 tbsp mango chutney

150g cooked lentils

1 apple, peeled and diced

small bunch of coriander, finely chopped

$\frac{1}{2}$ bunch of spring onions, cut into rounds (including the greens)

100g baby leaf spinach or similar greens

squeeze of lemon (optional)

salt and black pepper

Put the flaked almonds in a large frying pan or sauté pan and dry fry them, stirring constantly, until they are lightly golden. Keep a close eye on them, as they burn all too easily. Remove and set aside.

Heat the oil in the pan. Add the cauliflower and leave it for 3–4 minutes until the florets are brown or lightly charred on the underside. Turn them over and cook for a further 2–3 minutes, then add the curry powder.

Stir thoroughly for another minute, so the curry powder and the oil coat the cauliflower, then pour in 100ml of water. Season well, cover the pan and leave to steam for another 2–3 minutes. The cauliflower should still have a little bite to it. Stir in the mango chutney and then remove the pan from the heat.

Leave to cool for 5 minutes, then stir in the lentils, diced apple, half the coriander and the spring onions. Add the spinach and fold it in gently. Taste for seasoning, then add more salt as needed and a squeeze of lemon if you like. Sprinkle with the remaining coriander and serve.

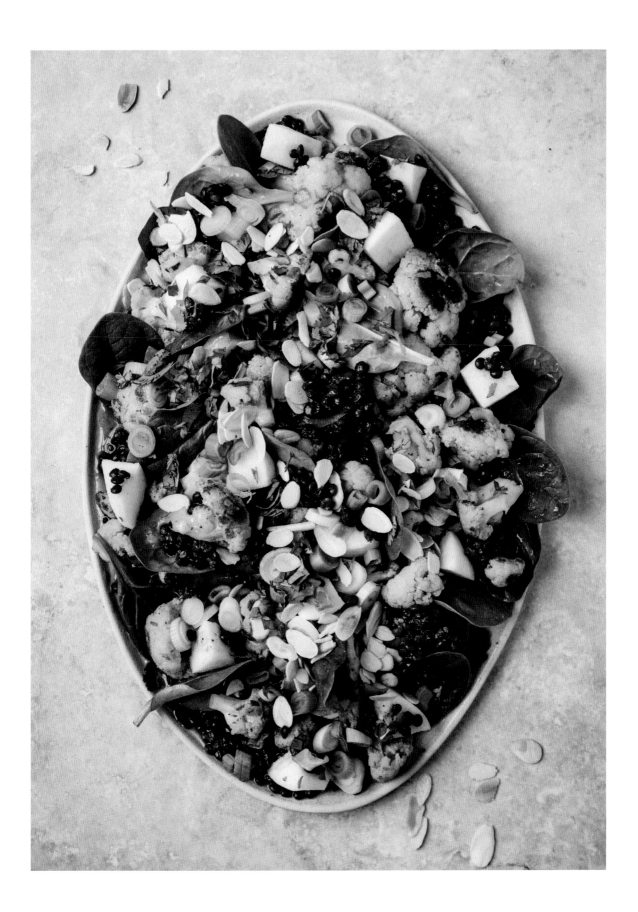

Hearty ham and cheese coleslaw

Kingy is a proper coleslaw monster and this recipe elevates his passion to a new level. You usually think of coleslaw as a side dish, but adding some ham and delicious smoked cheese makes this into a proper filling salad meal. And dead good it is too. We like to serve this on large lettuce leaves if we're feeling fancy.

Serves 4

½ medium white cabbage, shredded very finely

½ medium green cabbage, shredded very finely

1 large carrot, cut into thin matchsticks

1 onion, finely sliced

1 red or green chilli, finely chopped (optional)

1 tsp smoked chilli flakes (optional)

leaves from a small bunch of coriander, finely chopped

zest of 1 lime

100g ham, finely shredded

125g smoked cheese, grated

large iceberg lettuce leaves, to serve (optional)

salt and black pepper

Dressing
2 tbsp mayonnaise

2 tbsp buttermilk (see p.36)

1 tbsp cider vinegar

juice of ½ lime

½ tsp sugar

Put the white and green cabbage, the carrot and onion in a large colander and sprinkle with a heaped teaspoon of salt. Mix gently with your hands, then leave to stand in the sink for an hour. This will help the vegetables release some water and keep them nice and crisp.

Whisk the dressing ingredients together in a bowl large enough to hold the coleslaw and season with a little salt and pepper. Taste and adjust the sugar and vinegar to your liking – the dressing should taste pleasantly sharp, but not astringent.

Pat the contents of the colander dry and add them to the bowl of dressing, together with all the other ingredients. Mix thoroughly. Serve on large iceberg lettuce leaves, if you like, or in bowls.

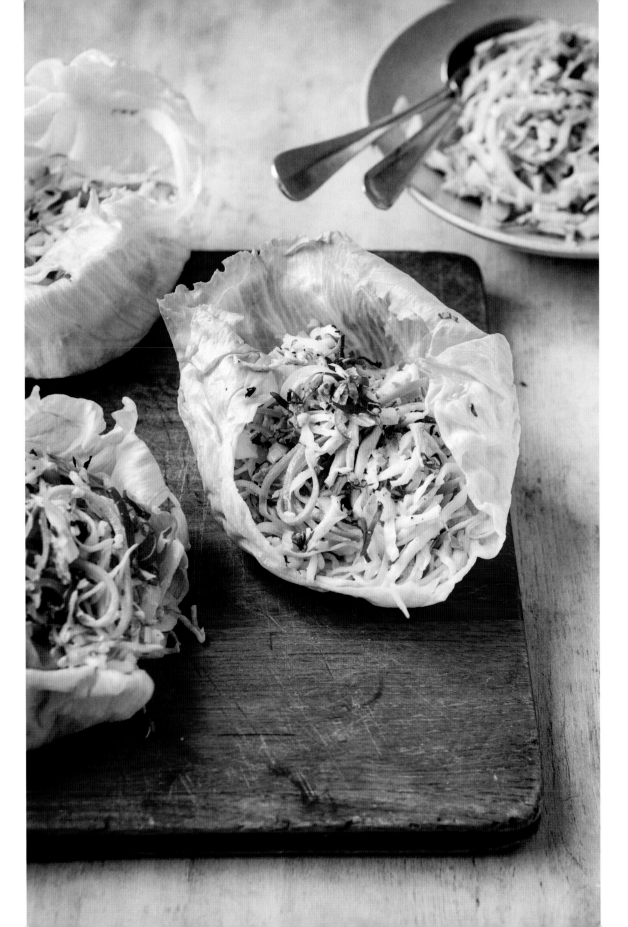

Our big Biker tabbouleh

Just 50g of bulgur is fine here – too much destroys the herby nature of this lovely dish and don't be frightened of going large with the herbs. We've made our version a little heartier by adding some chickpeas, cheese and a garnish of olives and pomegranate seeds. Hey presto, we have a main meal salad.

Serves 4

50g fine bulgur wheat

½ cucumber

400g can of chickpeas, drained and rinsed

bunch of spring onions, finely sliced

large bunch of parsley (at least 200g), very finely chopped

small bunch of mint (leaves only), very finely chopped

100g rocket, shredded

salt and black pepper

Garnish

50g black olives, finely chopped

seeds from ½ pomegranate

200g feta, finely diced (optional)

Dressing

4 tbsp olive oil

juice of 1 lemon

1 tbsp tahini

½ tsp ground allspice

½ tsp cinnamon

½ tsp ground coriander

First make the dressing. Put the olive oil, lemon juice, tahini and spices in a large salad bowl and season with salt and plenty of black pepper. Whisk together.

Rinse the bulgur wheat in cold water until it runs clear, then drain thoroughly. This is all the preparation that fine bulgur wheat needs. Add it to the salad bowl.

Peel, deseed and finely dice the cucumber and add it to the bowl with the chickpeas, spring onions, herbs and rocket. Pour over the dressing and stir everything together gently, but thoroughly, then taste for seasoning – add a little more lemon juice or salt and pepper if you think it needs it. Garnish with the olives, pomegranate seeds and feta, if using.

Succotash salad

Succotash is a favourite American dish that's often served as a side. There are lots of different versions but all contain sweetcorn. We've taken the basic idea and made it into a hearty salad.

Serves 4

3 tbsp olive oil

1 red onion, diced

100g okra, trimmed and sliced into rounds (optional)

250g sweetcorn, defrosted if frozen

400g can of butterbeans or black-eyed beans, drained and rinsed

1 red pepper, diced

200g cherry tomatoes, halved

1 heart of romaine/cos lettuce, shredded

200g ham, diced

1 tbsp sherry vinegar

handful of basil leaves, torn, to garnish

salt and black pepper

Heat the olive oil in a large frying pan. Add the onion and okra, if using, and cook over a medium heat for about 5 minutes, stirring regularly. Add the sweetcorn and continue to cook over a high heat, until the sweetcorn is lightly browned. Remove the pan from the heat and allow to cool.

Stir in the beans, red pepper, tomatoes, lettuce and ham. Drizzle over the sherry vinegar and season with plenty of salt and pepper. Transfer to a bowl if you like, garnish with the basil leaves and serve immediately.

Prawn, avocado and quinoa salad

Who doesn't love avocado and prawns?! We really got to like quinoa, too, when we were writing our Hairy Dieters books and now we often add some to our salads. It's rich in protein as well as filling, and it's a really good addition to this dish. You can buy ready-cooked quinoa which makes this salad super easy or cook some yourself.

Serves 4

2 tbsp olive oil

1 garlic clove, crushed

1 red chilli, finely chopped

juice and zest of 1 lime

pinch of curry powder

300g cooked, shelled tiger prawns

1 avocado, diced

250g cooked quinoa

150g rocket or mixed salad leaves

bunch of spring onions, sliced into rounds

bunch of coriander, roughly chopped

handful of mint leaves, roughly torn

¼–½ tsp smoked chilli flakes (or to taste)

salt and black pepper

Put the oil, garlic, chilli, lime juice and zest in a bowl with plenty of salt and pepper and the curry powder. Add the tiger prawns and avocado and toss gently to coat them in the seasonings. If you have time, leave everything to marinate for 20–30 minutes so the prawns can absorb all the flavours.

Sprinkle the quinoa over a large serving dish. Add the rocket or mixed salad leaves, followed by the spring onions, coriander and mint. Top with the contents of the bowl and toss very gently and briefly, then sprinkle with the chilli flakes. Serve immediately.

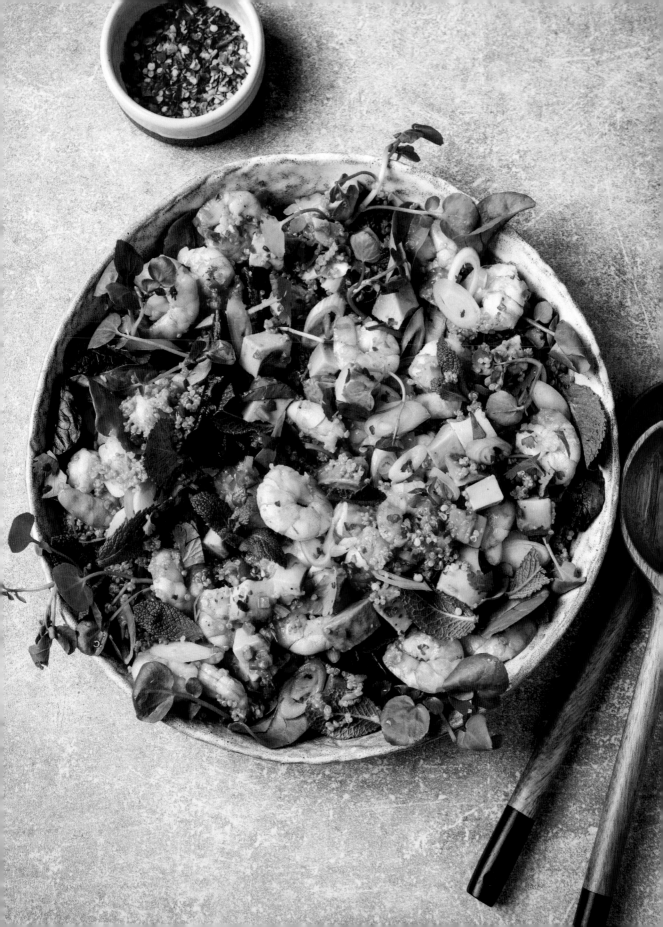

Spicy couscous salad

A doddle, this one. Just prepare the couscous in a big bowl, add everything else, then take it to the table and dig in. The only tricky bit is segmenting the oranges but once you get the idea you'll be doing it as easily as those chefs on Saturday Kitchen! And if there's any salad left over, pile it into a lunchbox to take to work with you the next day.

Serves 4

100g couscous

¼ tsp ground cinnamon

¼ tsp ground allspice

½ tsp dried oregano

120ml just-boiled water

2 oranges (see method)

2 medium tomatoes, diced

50g black olives, pitted and sliced

½ cucumber, deseeded and diced

100g goats' cheese

50g rocket, roughly chopped

large bunch of parsley, leaves only

small bunch of mint, leaves only

few sprigs of fresh oregano or marjoram, leaves only

2 tbsp olive oil

juice of ½ lemon

salt and black pepper

Pour the couscous into a large bowl and add the spices, a generous pinch of salt and pepper and the dried oregano. Pour over the just-boiled water and leave to stand until all the water is absorbed. Fluff up the couscous with a fork.

Next, prepare the oranges. Top and tail them, then stand them upright on a chopping board and cut away the flesh, following the curve of the orange. Squeeze the juice from the oranges into the couscous. Next, cut the segments out from the membrane – do this over the couscous to catch any juice. Break the orange segments up into small pieces and add them to the bowl. Squeeze the juice from the membrane into the bowl and discard the membrane.

Add the tomatoes, olives and cucumber to the couscous, and fold everything together. Crumble in the cheese and fold it in. Add the rocket and herbs, then drizzle over the olive oil and lemon juice. Check for seasoning (the olives will make the salad quite salty) and serve.

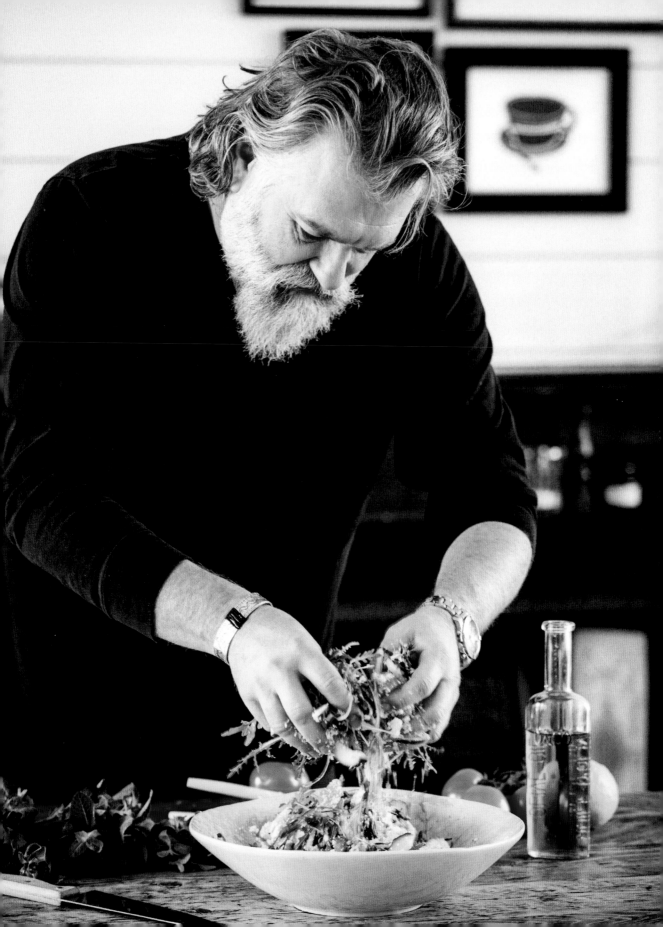

Panzanella

We did a frugal version of this called cialledda for our Mediterranean book, but now we've fired up the throttles. Here's our recipe for a classic Italian salad that began as a way of using up yesterday's bread, then turned into something super delicious. This conjures up visions of sunny lunches in a beachside café somewhere on the Mediterranean coast of Italy. Wish you were there?

Serves 4

2 red peppers, halved

200g ciabatta bread, or good sourdough, torn into chunks

2 tbsp olive oil

2 garlic cloves, crushed

1 red onion, thinly sliced

300g ripe tomatoes

50g can of anchovies

2 tbsp sherry vinegar

1 tbsp capers, roughly chopped

2 tbsp black olives, pitted and sliced

1 tsp dried oregano

bunch of basil

salt and black pepper

Preheat the oven to 200°C/Fan 180°C/Gas 6. Put the peppers in a roasting tin and roast until the skins have started to blacken – this takes about 15 minutes. Remove from the oven, put them in a plastic bag and leave to cool. Put the bread in the same tin, add the olive oil, garlic and plenty of seasoning and mix thoroughly. Roast for 10 minutes until the bread has crisped up a bit and turned golden brown.

While you are roasting the peppers and bread, sprinkle the red onion with salt and cover with water. Leave to stand for half an hour, then drain thoroughly.

Roughly chop the tomatoes and put them in a sieve. Sprinkle over plenty of salt and leave to drain over your salad bowl to catch the juice. Peel the peppers when they are cool enough to handle and tear them into strips.

Chop the anchovies finely and put them and their oil into the bowl. Add the sherry vinegar, capers and olives, then the bread. Mix thoroughly, so the bread is well coated, then add the chopped tomatoes, drained onion, pepper strips and the oregano and basil. Leave the salad to stand at room temperature for at least half an hour before serving.

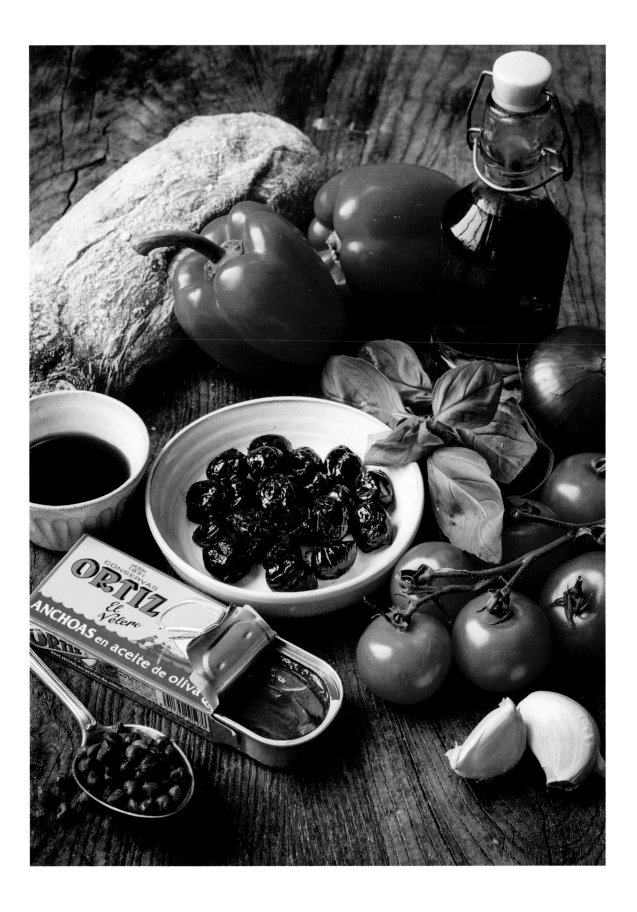

Chopped chicken salad

This makes a great dish for a summer lunch with friends. You can get everything more or less ready earlier in the day, then add the salad leaves just before sitting down to eat. A dead tasty bowlful, though we say it ourselves, and so easy to make with ready-cooked chicken.

Serves 4

2 cooked chicken breasts, diced

3 celery sticks, diced

bunch of spring onions, sliced into rounds

½ cucumber, deseeded and diced

100g radishes, thinly sliced

200g cherry tomatoes, halved

2 tarragon sprigs, finely chopped

2 thyme sprigs, leaves only

1 heart of romaine lettuce, finely chopped

50g watercress, stems finely chopped, leaves left whole

50g rocket, roughly chopped

50g Parmesan cheese, grated (optional)

Dressing
4 tbsp olive oil

1 tbsp sherry vinegar

1 tsp Dijon mustard

½ tsp runny honey

1 garlic clove, crushed

salt and black pepper

First make the dressing in your salad bowl. Whisk everything together with plenty of salt and pepper. Taste and add a little more honey, vinegar or seasoning to your liking.

Add the chicken to the bowl and toss so it is all well coated with dressing. Fold in the celery, spring onions, cucumber, radishes and cherry tomatoes, then the herbs. Stir everything together and season with salt and pepper. At this point, you can leave the salad until you are ready to serve it.

Just before serving, add the lettuce, watercress and rocket. Add the Parmesan, if using, for some extra richness and toss this through too. Eat at once.

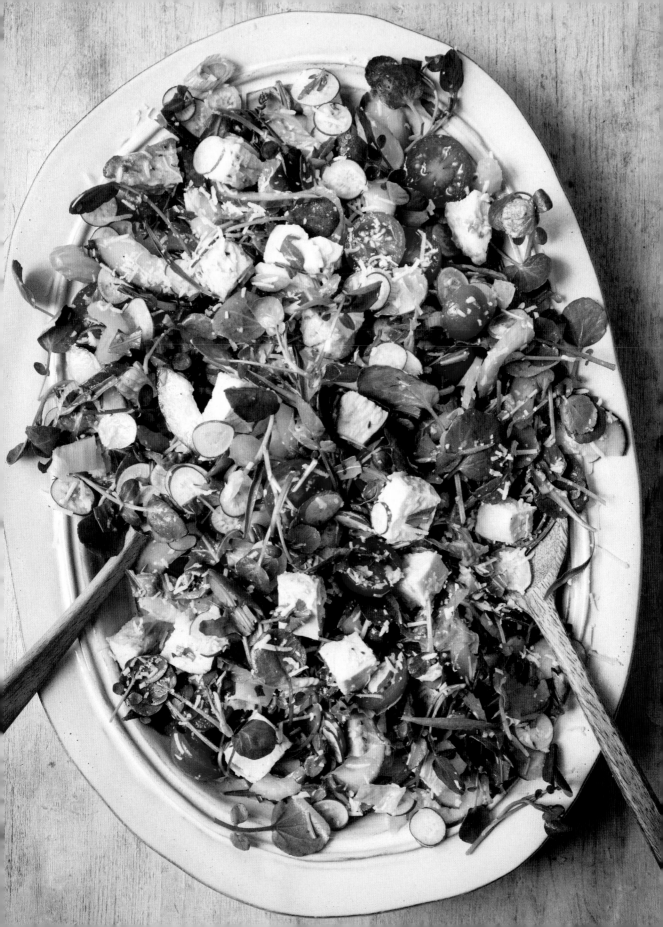

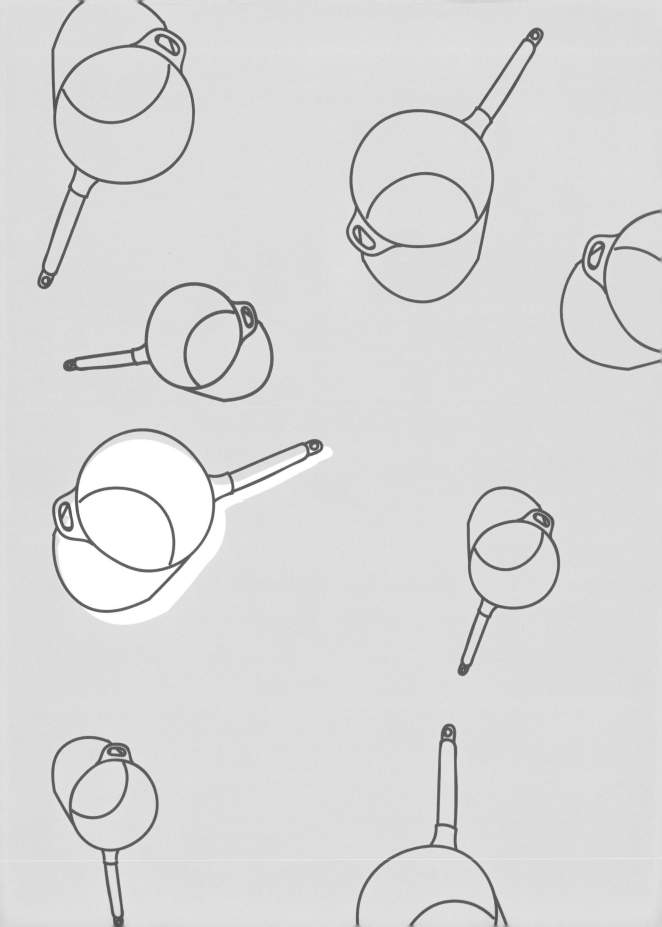

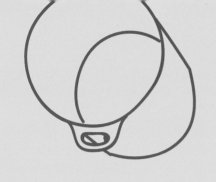

Satisfying Soups and Stews

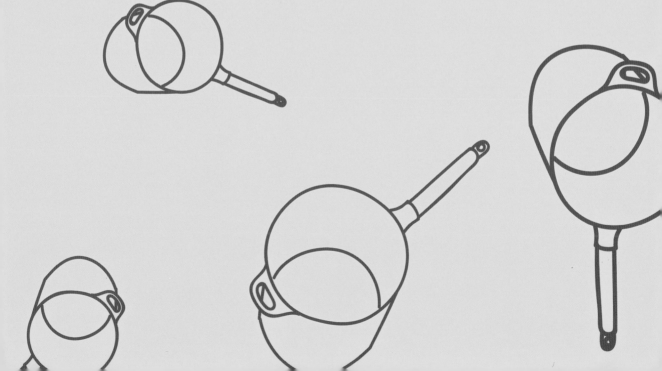

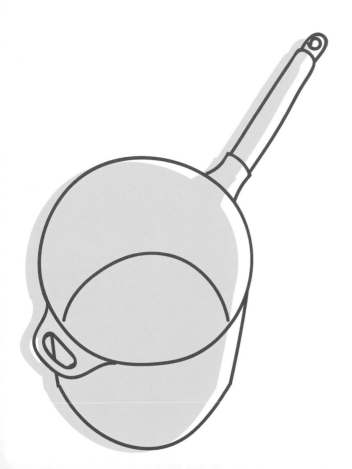

Broccoli and cheese soup

One of our favourite veg, broccoli makes an excellent soup and adding cheese means that this is filling and nourishing too. A bowlful of goodness, and if you want a vegetarian soup, just leave out the bacon.

Serves 4

2 tbsp olive oil

4 slices of streaky bacon, very finely chopped (optional)

1 onion, finely chopped

2 celery sticks, finely chopped

1 large floury potato, finely diced

2 garlic cloves, crushed

800ml vegetable or chicken stock

500g broccoli, roughly chopped

125g mature Cheddar cheese, grated

1 tbsp wholegrain mustard (optional)

salt and black pepper

To serve
single cream

Heat the oil in a large pan. Add the bacon, if using, and fry until it's crisp and brown and some fat has rendered out. Remove the bacon from the pan with a slotted spoon and set aside.

Add the onion, celery and potato to the pan and cook until the onion is soft and translucent. Then add the garlic, followed by the stock, and season with salt and pepper. Bring to the boil, then turn the heat down to a simmer. Add the broccoli and simmer until all the vegetables are tender.

Using a stick blender, blitz the soup until smooth, then stir in the cheese and the mustard, if using. Serve the soup piping hot, topped with the bacon, if using, and a generous swirl of cream.

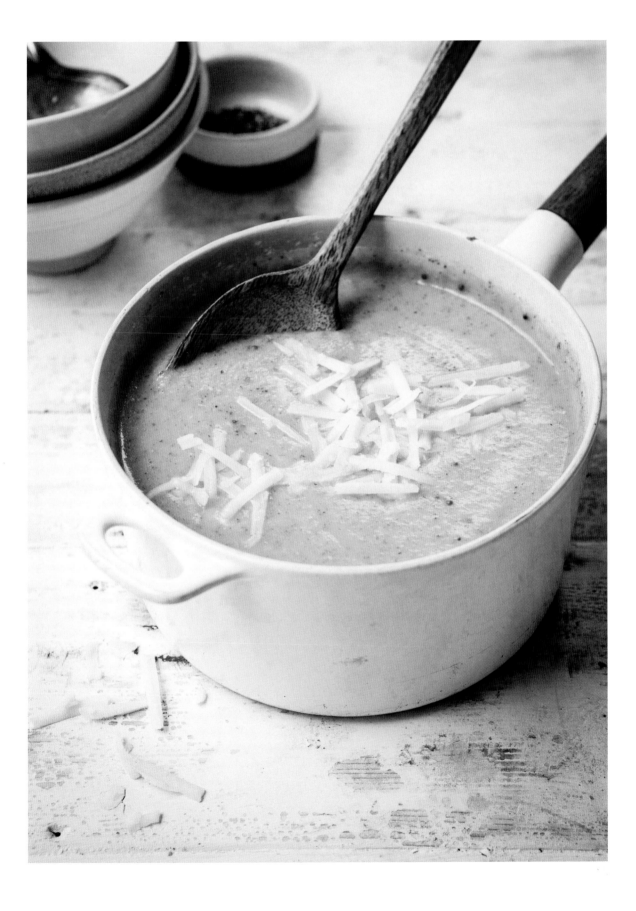

Tomato and watermelon gazpacho

A one pot that doesn't even need a pot – this is just whizzed up in a blender and it's done. Plenty of time for you and the soup to chill before eating. The watermelon works brilliantly to add freshness to this, the most summery soup imaginable.

Serves 4

400g ripe tomatoes

300g watermelon, deseeded and cut into chunks

½ cucumber, peeled

½ red pepper, diced

2 celery sticks, roughly chopped

3 spring onions, sliced

2 garlic cloves, chopped

handful of basil leaves

75g stale white bread

1 tsp smoked chilli flakes or 1–2 tsp chilli paste

1 tbsp sherry vinegar

2 tbsp olive oil

salt and black pepper

To garnish

juice of ½ lime

1 avocado, finely diced

fresh coriander

Put all the soup ingredients into a blender with plenty of salt and pepper. Blitz until smooth, but if the soup isn't smooth enough for your liking, push it through a sieve.

Taste the soup for seasoning and add more salt, pepper or vinegar if you think it needs it. Chill thoroughly in the fridge – this is best served ice cold.

Mix the lime juice with the avocado and plenty of salt. Serve the soup garnished with the avocado and some fresh coriander.

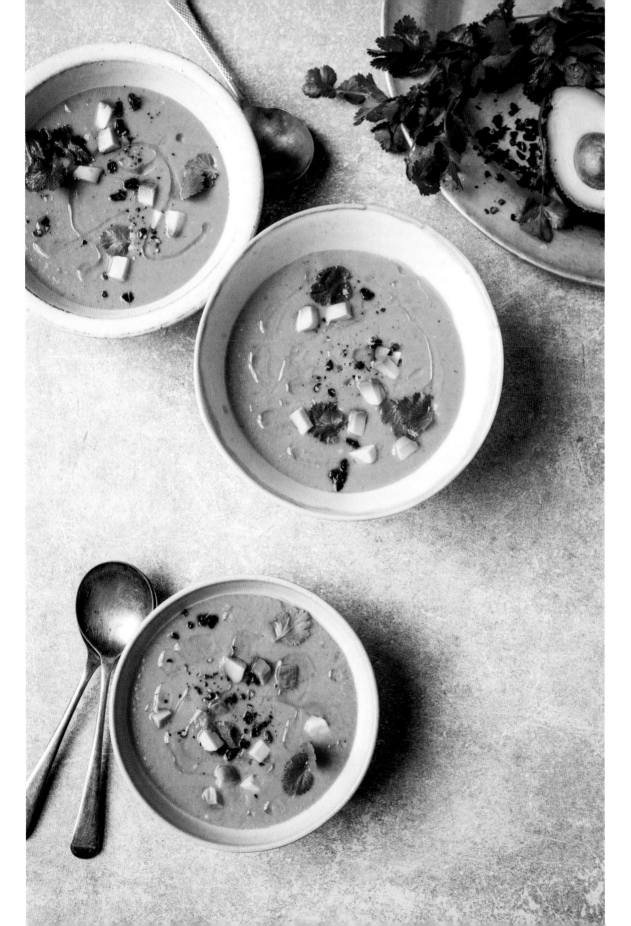

Austrian garlic soup

We discovered this soup when we were filming *Bakeation* in Austria years ago. It's quick to make and so warming and good. It's quite rich so you don't need a lot, and the crunchy croutons are the perfect finishing touch. Simply addictive.

Serves 4

50g butter

10 fat garlic cloves, crushed or grated

25g flour

250ml milk

500ml chicken or vegetable stock

2 tbsp white wine

salt and black pepper

To serve

2 thick slices of robust bread

1 garlic clove, halved

finely chopped parsley

Melt the butter in a saucepan. When it's foaming, add the garlic and season with plenty of salt and pepper. Cook for several minutes over a low to medium heat until the garlic smells much more intense and it has started to separate from the butter. Stir the garlic while it cooks and don't let it start to brown.

Add the flour and stir for a few more minutes to make sure its raw flavour has been cooked out. Start adding the milk, then the stock, a little at a time, stirring constantly. By the time you have incorporated all the liquid, you should have a thin soup that is about the consistency of unwhipped cream. Add the wine and simmer the soup gently for another 10 minutes to mellow the flavour of the garlic and wine.

Toast the slices of bread and rub them with the garlic halves, then cut them into croutons. Stir the parsley into the soup and serve with the croutons.

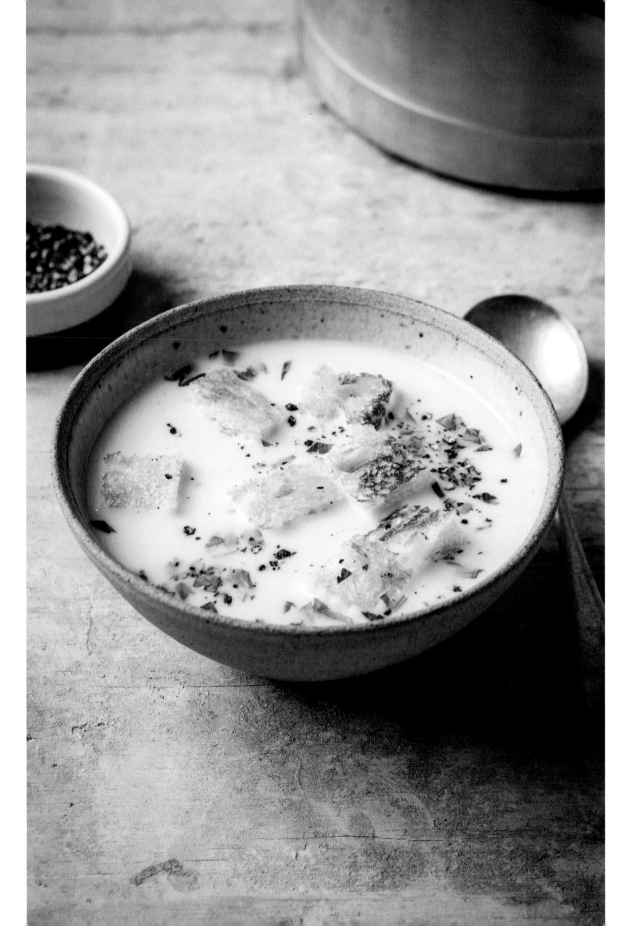

Pea and watercress soup

The short cooking time means that this soup stays lovely and fresh and green. The peppery watercress goes perfectly with the sweetness of the peas and we think it lifts the spirits just to look at it! Springtime in a bowl.

Serves 4

1 tbsp olive oil

15g butter

2 leeks, finely diced

1 garlic clove, finely chopped

small bunch of fresh mint, leaves only, or 1 tsp dried mint

150g watercress, roughly chopped

800ml vegetable or chicken stock

500g frozen peas

salt and black pepper

To serve
single cream
mint leaves

Heat the oil and butter in a large pan. When the butter has melted, add the leeks and cook them over a low heat for several minutes until soft and glossy. Add the garlic and cook for 2 minutes longer.

Add the mint leaves or dried mint to the pan, together with the watercress. Stir until the watercress has wilted down, then pour in the stock. Add the peas and season with salt and pepper, then bring to the boil. Turn down the heat and simmer for 3–4 minutes.

Remove the soup from the heat and blitz with a hand-held blender – you can make it completely smooth or, better still, leave it flecked with green. Reheat gently and serve immediately with a swirl of cream and a few mint leaves.

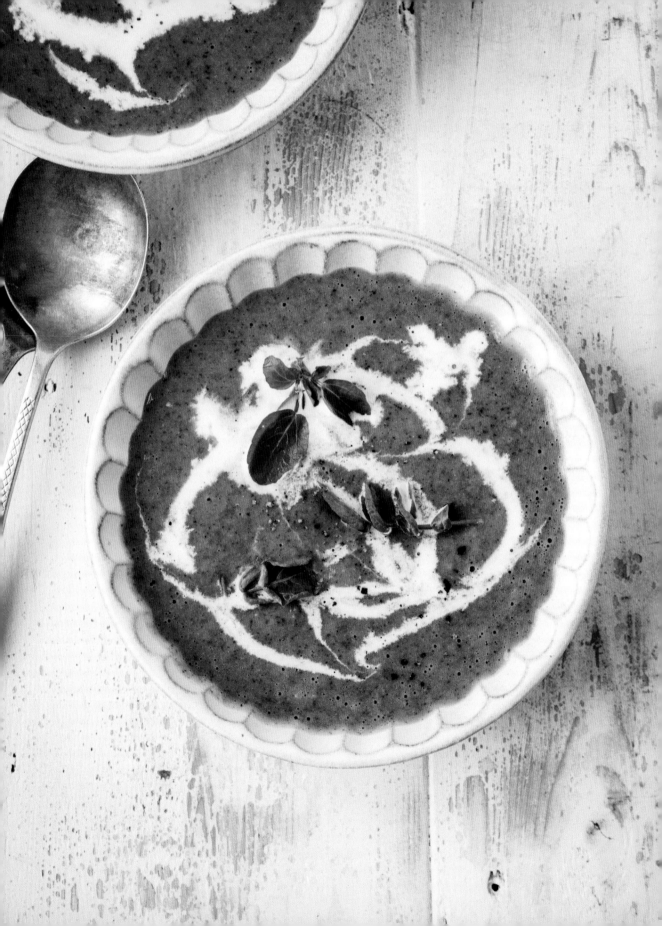

Summery minestrone

You can't go wrong with a good minestrone and this one is packed full of summery veg. We've suggested adding a Parmesan cheese rind if you have one – that's the little lumpy bit left when you can't grate it any more – as it does add great flavour. And the crowning glory is a swirl of pesto. Shop-bought is fine or you'll find a recipe on page 271.

Serves 4

2 tbsp olive oil

3 leeks, sliced on the diagonal

3 courgettes, sliced on the diagonal

200g runner beans, trimmed and cut into strips

2 garlic cloves, finely chopped

2 tarragon sprigs

1 parsley sprig

2 bay leaves

1 piece of pared lemon zest

1 litre vegetable or chicken stock

Parmesan rind (optional)

100g broad beans (fresh or frozen)

3 little gem lettuces, quartered into wedges

400g can of cannellini beans, drained and rinsed

salt and black pepper

To serve
basil leaves (optional)
mint leaves (optional)
basil pesto

Heat the oil in a large saucepan. Add the leeks and cook them over a medium to low heat until they are starting to soften. Add the courgettes, runner beans, garlic, herbs and lemon zest and cook for another 3–4 minutes.

Pour in the stock and season with salt and pepper. If you have a Parmesan rind, add it now – some of it will dissolve into the stock and provide extra flavour. Bring the soup to the boil, then turn the heat down and simmer, uncovered, until the vegetables are just tender. Add the broad beans and little gems and continue to cook until the little gems have wilted and their cores are tender.

Add the cannellini beans and heat them through. Fish out the remains of the Parmesan rind, the sprigs of herbs and the bay leaves. Serve the soup garnished with basil and mint leaves, if using, and spoonfuls of pesto.

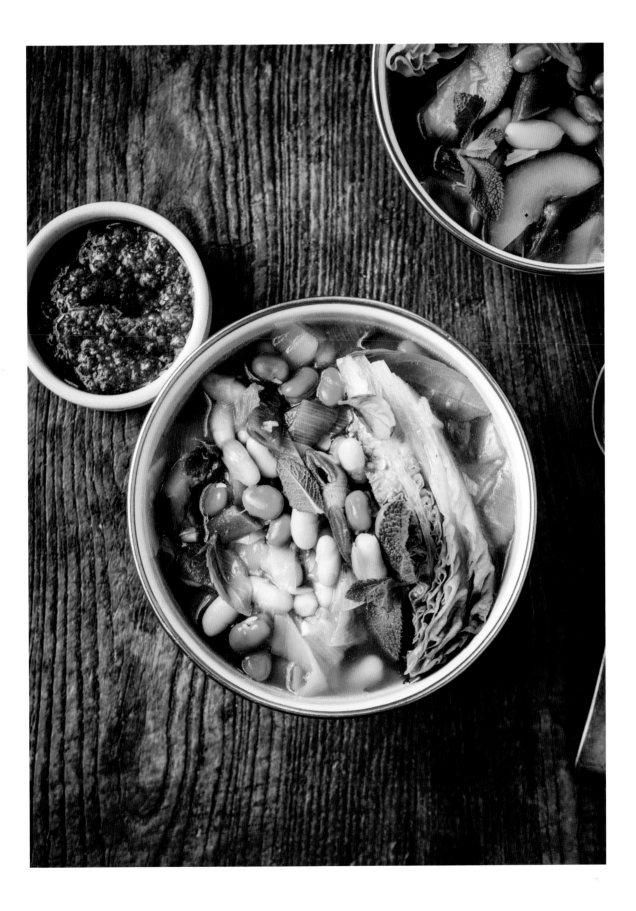

Smoky fish chowder

There's nothing as warming and comforting as a bowl of fish chowder. This was inspired by a frugal dish called cullen skink that we cooked a long while back, but this recipe is bang up to date, with a hint of luxury. We decided not to add bacon, as the smoked haddock gives that nice smoky flavour.

Serves 4

25g butter

1 onion, finely diced

2 leeks, cut into rounds

2 floury potatoes, peeled and diced

1 garlic clove, chopped

2 tarragon sprigs

1 bay leaf

100ml white wine

750ml milk

150g sweetcorn (frozen is fine)

300g white fish, skinned and cut into chunks

200g smoked haddock, skinned and cut into chunks

100ml double cream

salt and black pepper

To serve
finely snipped chives

Heat the butter in a large saucepan and add the onion, leeks and potatoes. Cook over a low heat for several minutes until the onion is starting to look soft and translucent, then add the garlic, tarragon and bay leaf. Stir for a couple more minutes, then turn up the heat and add the wine. Bring to the boil and let most of the wine boil away.

Season with salt and pepper and pour in the milk, then turn up the heat again. When the soup is close to boiling point, turn down the heat and simmer until the vegetables are tender. Mash the potatoes very lightly just to break them down a little so they help thicken the soup.

Add the sweetcorn and the white fish and smoked haddock. Continue to simmer until the fish is cooked through – this should take 3–4 minutes. Stir in the double cream and heat it through. Garnish with plenty of chives and serve at once.

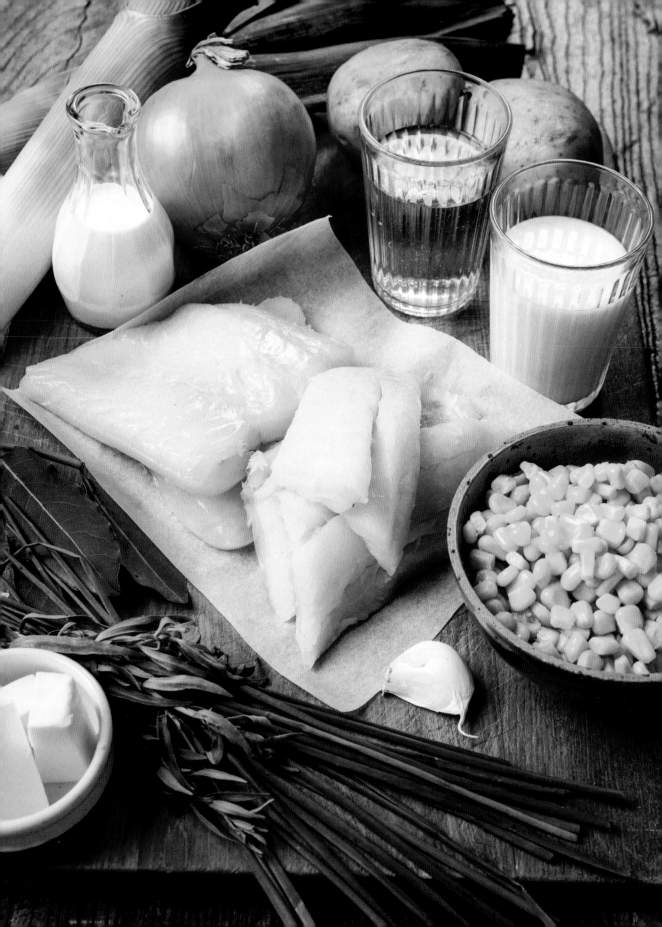

Spicy lentil and kale soup

We've gone a bit Moroccan with this soup and added a good dollop of spicy harissa paste to give it a real punch. You can buy good harissa paste in supermarkets or if you fancy making your own, have a look at our recipe on page 270. This will keep you regular – regularly coming back for a second bowlful.

Serves 4

2 tbsp olive oil

1 onion, finely chopped

1 carrot, finely chopped

2 celery sticks, finely chopped

2 tbsp red harissa paste

200g brown lentils

1.5 litres vegetable stock
   or water

200g kale or spinach

salt and black pepper

To serve
squeeze of lemon

finely chopped parsley

Heat the oil in a large pan and add the onion, carrot and celery. Cook for about 10 minutes over a medium to low heat, until the vegetables have started to soften and brown slightly around the edges.

Stir in the harissa paste, followed by the lentils and season with salt and pepper. Pour over the stock or water and bring to the boil. Partially cover the pan and leave to simmer until the lentils are tender and have started to collapse into the soup. This should take 20–30 minutes.

If you're using kale, cut out any thick woody stems, shred the leaves and add them to the soup after the lentils have been cooking for 20 minutes. If you're using spinach, add it once the lentils are cooked.

You can leave the soup as it is if you like the texture, or blitz it with a stick blender to break it down further. Serve with a squeeze of lemon juice and a sprinkling of parsley.

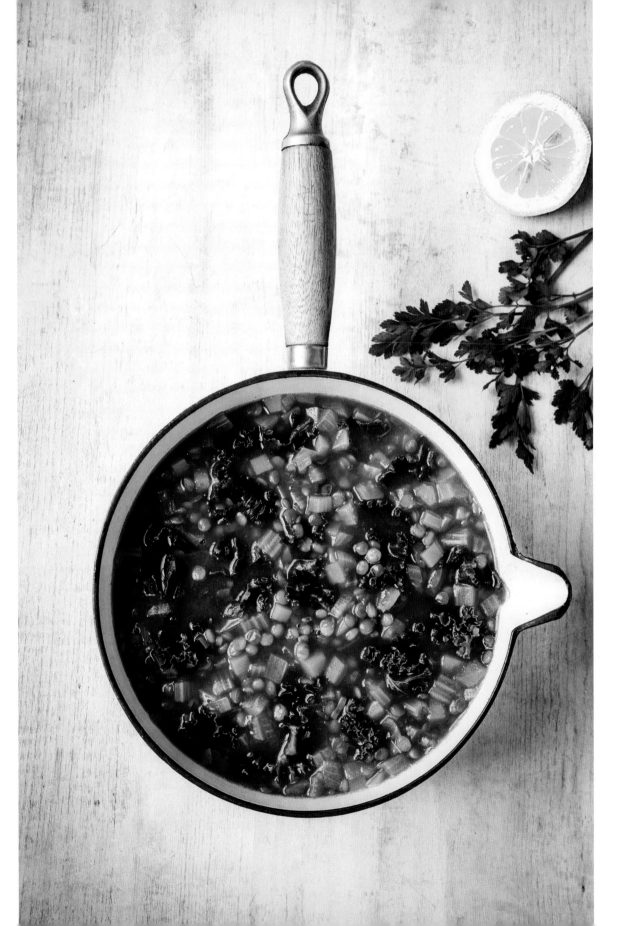

Quick prawn laksa

This is a quick and easy version of laksa, using shop-bought paste for speed, but if you do want to make your own there's a recipe on page 269. Packed full of great flavours, this is one of our favourite soups.

Serves 4

1 tbsp vegetable oil
200g raw shelled prawns
2 tbsp laksa paste
750ml fish or chicken stock
400ml can of coconut milk
1 tbsp fish sauce
2 Kaffir lime leaves, shredded
handful of Chinese greens
250g firm-fleshed white fish,
    cut into chunks
salt and black pepper

To serve
400g cooked rice noodles
½ bunch of spring onions,
halved and shredded
chopped fresh coriander
a few mint leaves
lime wedges

Heat the oil in a large flameproof casserole dish or a saucepan. Add the prawns and sear them on both sides, then remove them and set aside. Add the laksa paste and fry for a few minutes until it smells very aromatic and the oil has started to separate from the paste – you will see small droplets of bright orange oil form.

Pour in the stock and coconut milk, then add the fish sauce and lime leaves. Bring to the boil, then turn the heat down and taste – add salt and pepper if needed. Simmer for 25–30 minutes until the sauce has reduced down a bit and is about the consistency of single cream.

Add the greens, then the fish and simmer for another 3–4 minutes, until the fish is cooked. Put the prawns back in the pan to heat through. To serve, divide the noodles between your bowls, ladle over the laksa and garnish with spring onions, coriander and mint leaves. Provide lime wedges for squeezing over.

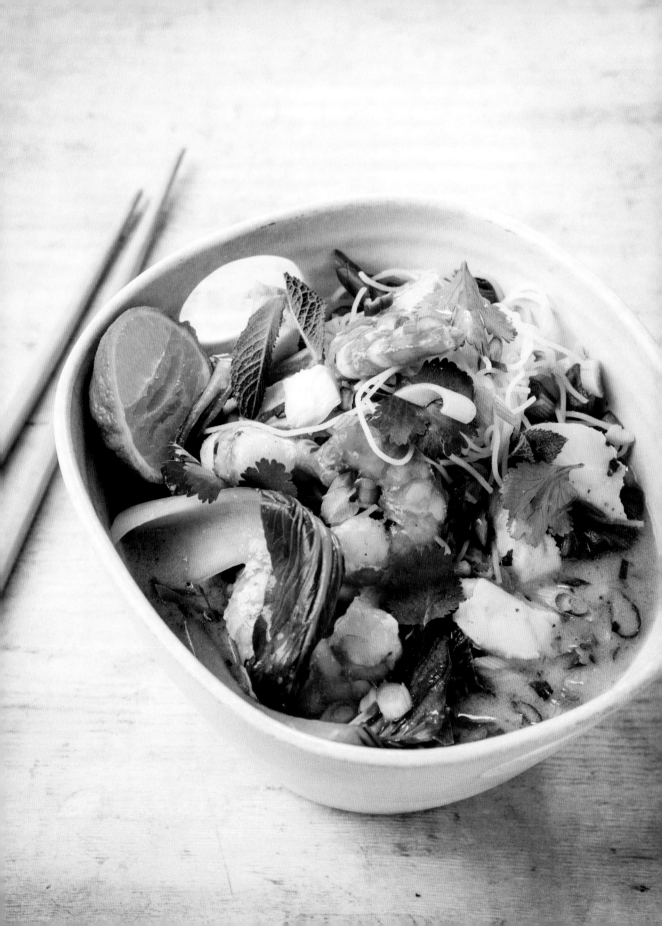

Chicken, lemon and orzo soup

Chicken and lemon soup has always been a classic and this one is no exception – another great main meal soup. Orzo is actually a type of pasta, cut into tiny pieces about the size of a grain of rice, and it's perfect for adding to soup. This dish is also good served cold, but if you do want to reheat it, take care not to let it boil or it will curdle.

Serves 4

25g butter

1 onion, finely sliced

2 skinless, boneless chicken breasts, finely diced

2 garlic cloves, finely chopped

2 bay leaves

75g orzo

1 litre chicken stock

3 eggs

juice of 1 lemon

salt and black pepper

To serve
a few dill fronds

Heat the butter in a large pan. When it has melted, add the onion and cook it gently until soft and translucent. Add the diced chicken breasts and cook them gently too – they should remain pale in colour. Add the garlic and cook for a couple more minutes, then season with salt and pepper.

Stir in the bay leaves and the orzo, then pour over the stock. Bring the soup to the boil, then turn the heat down and simmer until the orzo is cooked through and the onion is very tender.

Whisk the eggs until very smooth – put them through a sieve to be sure. Add the lemon juice and continue to whisk, then take a ladleful of the chicken broth and pour it into the bowl of eggs from a height, whisking continually. Gradually stir this mixture back into the soup, making sure you do not let it boil – it will curdle if you do. After a few minutes of stirring, the soup will thicken slightly and take on a smooth, silky texture.

Serve garnished with fronds of dill.

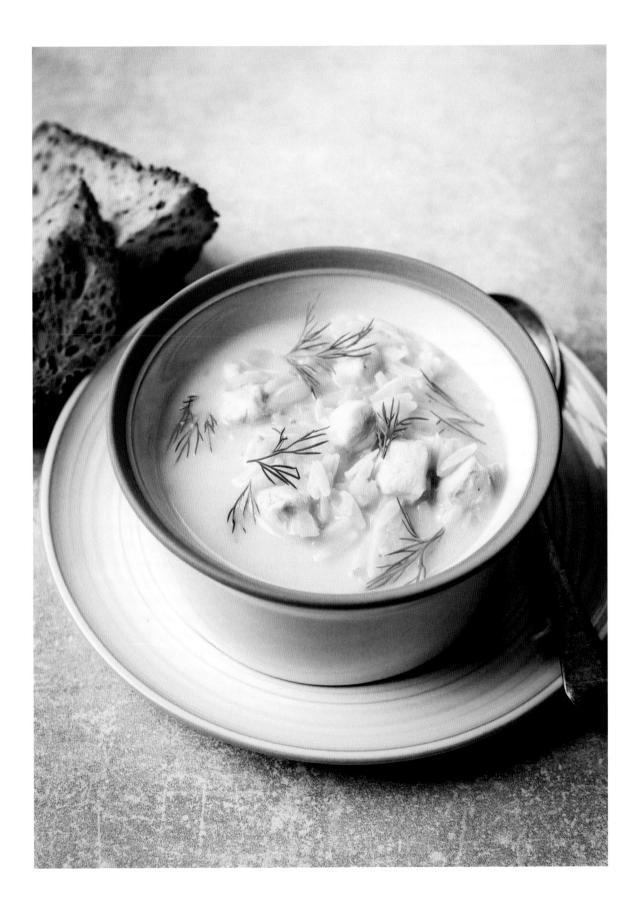

Lamb, barley and spring greens soup

A good hearty soup this one and the lamb and barley work so well together. We like to add chopped mint at the end to bring some nice freshness, but you could use parsley instead if you prefer. A proper pot au fabulous, we think.

Serves 4

2 tbsp olive oil

1 large onion, diced

2 carrots, diced

3 celery sticks, diced

1 leek, finely sliced

1 large potato, diced

200g butternut squash or similar, diced

300g lean lamb, finely diced

a few rosemary sprigs

a large thyme sprig

$\frac{1}{2}$ tsp rubbed sage

3 garlic cloves, chopped

50g pearl barley

1.5 litres lamb stock or water

about 150g spring greens, shredded

salt and black pepper

To serve
chopped mint leaves

Heat the oil in a large pan. Add the onion, carrots, celery, leek, potato and squash. Cook over a high heat until the vegetables are starting to caramelise around the edges, then add the lamb. Stir until it is browned all over, then add the herbs, garlic and barley. Stir for another minute until the barley looks glossy.

Season well with salt and pepper and then pour in the stock or water. Bring to the boil, then turn down the heat to a simmer and cook for at least an hour until the vegetables are tender and the barley is cooked but still has a slight bite to it. Add the greens and push them down into the liquid. Simmer for another 10 minutes until the greens are cooked through, then sprinkle with the chopped mint and serve.

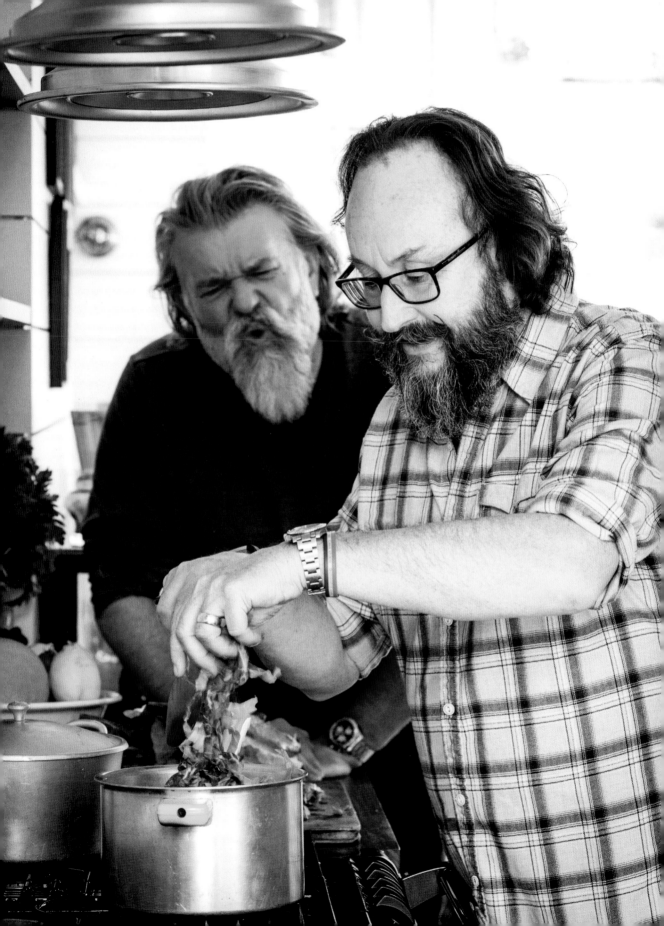

Hot and sour Thai chicken soup

Okay, we know there's quite a long list of stuff here, but several things are used both for the broth and the soup so it's not as bad as it looks. Also, some supermarkets sell little kits of Thai ingredients, which makes the shopping easier. And once you have everything ready, this is quick to make – and well worth it. A great wake-you-up soup.

Serves 4

Broth

1 litre chicken stock

½ tsp light soft brown sugar

2 lemongrass stalks, bruised

10g galangal, sliced

10g fresh root ginger, sliced

4 Kaffir lime leaves

2 skinless, boneless chicken
   breasts

salt and black pepper

Soup

2–3 tbsp fish sauce

juice of 1 lime

white part of a lemongrass
   stalk, finely sliced

2 garlic cloves, sliced

4 Kaffir lime leaves, finely
   sliced

2–4 bird's eye chillies, sliced

100g salad potatoes, sliced

1 red pepper, thinly sliced

100g mangetout or sugar snap
   peas

100g sprouting broccoli, sliced
   lengthways

100g baby corn, halved
   lengthways

To serve

bunch of spring onions,
   finely sliced

chopped fresh coriander

First heat the stock in a large saucepan. Add plenty of salt and pepper, then the sugar, lemongrass, galangal, ginger and lime leaves. Bring to the boil, then add the chicken breasts. Simmer them over a low heat for 7–8 minutes until they are just cooked through, then remove them from the broth and set aside to cool. Leave the broth to cool and infuse, then strain it and discard all the solids. Pour the broth back into the pan.

When the chicken breasts are cool enough to handle, shred them or pull them apart. Add all the soup ingredients to the pan and bring to the boil, then turn down the heat and simmer until the potatoes are cooked. Add the chicken to the pan to heat through at the last minute.

Taste and adjust the seasoning, adding more fish sauce and lime juice if you think it necessary. Serve the soup garnished with plenty of spring onions and chopped coriander.

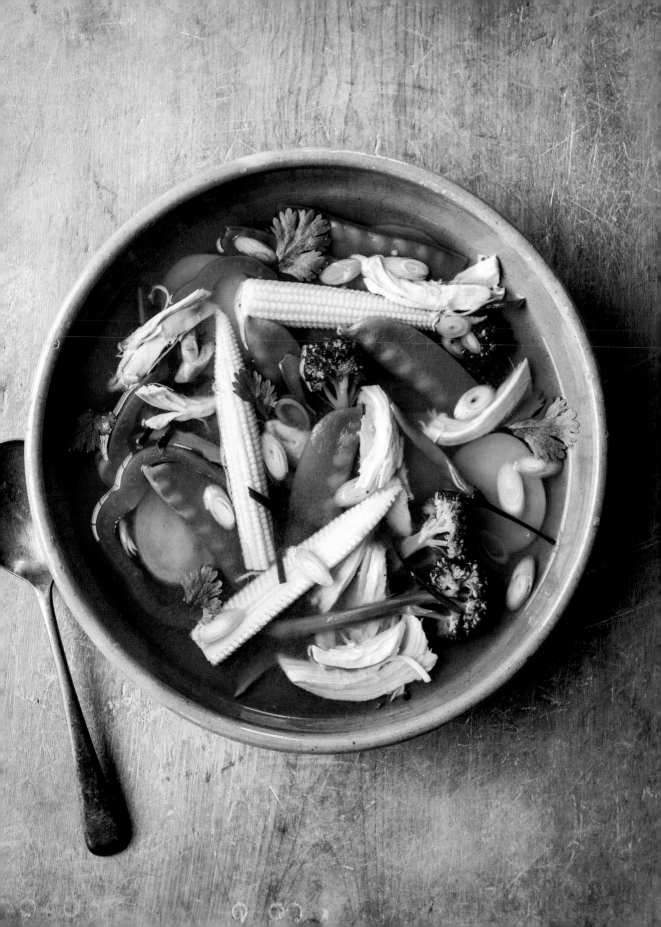

West Indian chicken curry with spinners

Spinners are the Jamaican version of dumplings and they have a denser texture than the regular sort. The idea is that they sink and spin as they cook, rather than bob around on the top of the dish – hence the name. Whatever they do, they're good to eat and just right with this curry.

Serves 4–6

2 tbsp vegetable or olive oil

1 large onion, chopped

1 large carrot, sliced into rounds

3 garlic cloves, finely chopped

10g fresh root ginger, grated

1–2 tbsp West Indian curry powder (shop-bought or see p.268)

6 boneless, skinless chicken thighs, diced

1 scotch bonnet chilli, left whole

large thyme sprig

400ml chicken stock

400ml coconut milk

1 tbsp tamarind purée

1 aubergine, diced

200g pumpkin, diced

1 tbsp sherry

1 lime, to serve

salt and black pepper

Spinners
125g plain flour

50g fine cornmeal

1 tsp vegetable oil

Heat the oil in a large flameproof casserole dish. Add the onion and carrot and cook for about 10 minutes until the onion is starting to soften. Add the garlic, ginger and curry powder and stir them in, then add the chicken and stir until it is completely coated in the oil and spices.

Season well with salt and pepper, then add the scotch bonnet and thyme to the casserole dish. Pour in the stock and coconut milk, then bring to the boil. Stir in the tamarind purée, then turn down the heat and simmer for 15 minutes, until the carrot is just tender. Add the aubergine and pumpkin, then continue to simmer until they're tender too – about another 15 minutes.

Make the spinners. Mix the flour and cornmeal with the oil and some salt, then work in 100ml of water until you have a firm, non-sticky dough. Divide this into 12 pieces, then roll each one into a log and twist the ends so they become more tapered. Drop the spinners into the curry and cook for 10–15 minutes until they are done.

Stir in the sherry and eat the curry with a squeeze of lime juice.

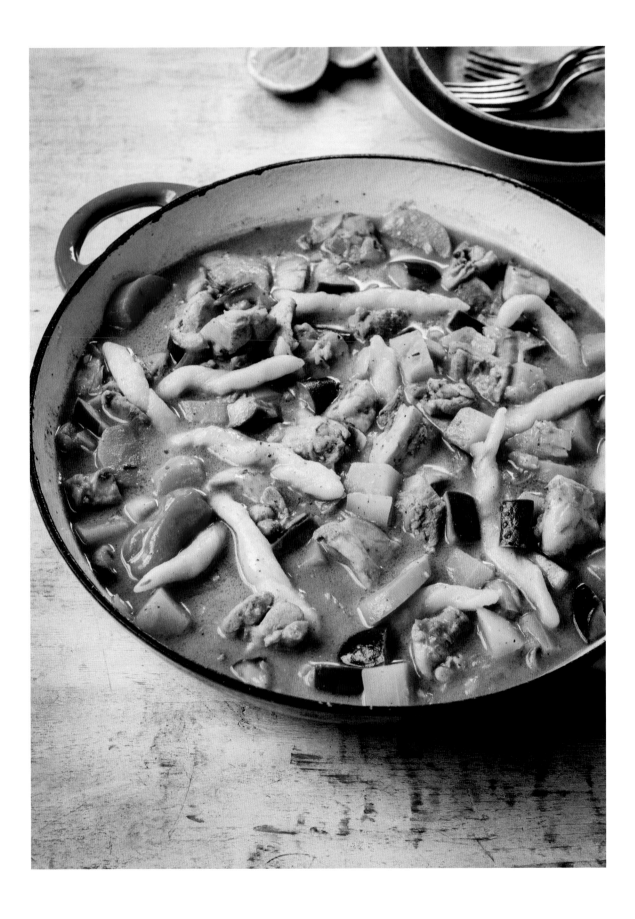

Rich oxtail stew

A good pot of oxtail stew was a regular in both our households when we were kids and we still love it today. We used to have it with mash but we've added some sweet potato to this recipe, so you have everything you need for a hearty meal. And if you've got any leftovers, strip off the meat, mix it with any juices and use it as a fantastic pasta sauce.

Serves 4–6

2kg oxtail pieces

50g plain flour

4 tbsp olive oil

1 onion, diced

1 large carrot, diced

2 celery sticks, diced

4 garlic cloves, finely chopped

1 red chilli, finely chopped

1 tbsp light soft brown sugar

1 tsp ground allspice

2 tbsp tomato purée

300ml red wine

bouquet garni (1 thyme sprig, 2 bay leaves and 2 parsley sprigs)

400ml beef stock

1 large sweet potato, peeled and cut into chunks

salt and black pepper

Trim the oxtail of any thick, hard pieces of fat, then pat the pieces dry. Dust the oxtail in the flour, brushing off any excess.

Heat half the olive oil in a large flameproof casserole dish, then fry the oxtail, a few pieces at a time, until they are all well seared. Set the oxtail aside, then add the onion, carrot and celery to the dish. Cook over a high heat until the vegetables have taken on some colour, then stir in the garlic and chilli. Cook for another couple of minutes, then stir in the sugar and allspice. Keep stirring until the sugar has dissolved, then add the tomato purée. Stir for another minute.

Pour in the red wine and bring to the boil. Season with plenty of salt and pepper, then put the oxtail back in the casserole. dish. Tuck in the bouquet garni and pour in the beef stock. Bring to the boil again, then turn down the heat and cover the pan. Leave the stew to simmer for at least 3 hours until the oxtail is tender but not quite falling off the bone.

Remove the oxtail from the casserole dish, followed by the vegetables – this is easily done with a slotted spoon. Leave the remaining liquid to cool. This makes the next job of removing the fat much easier, as it will collect on the top and set. Skim the fat off, then put the oxtail and vegetables back in the dish.

Add the sweet potato and bring the stew back to the boil. Simmer uncovered until the sauce has reduced down and the sweet potato is tender, then serve.

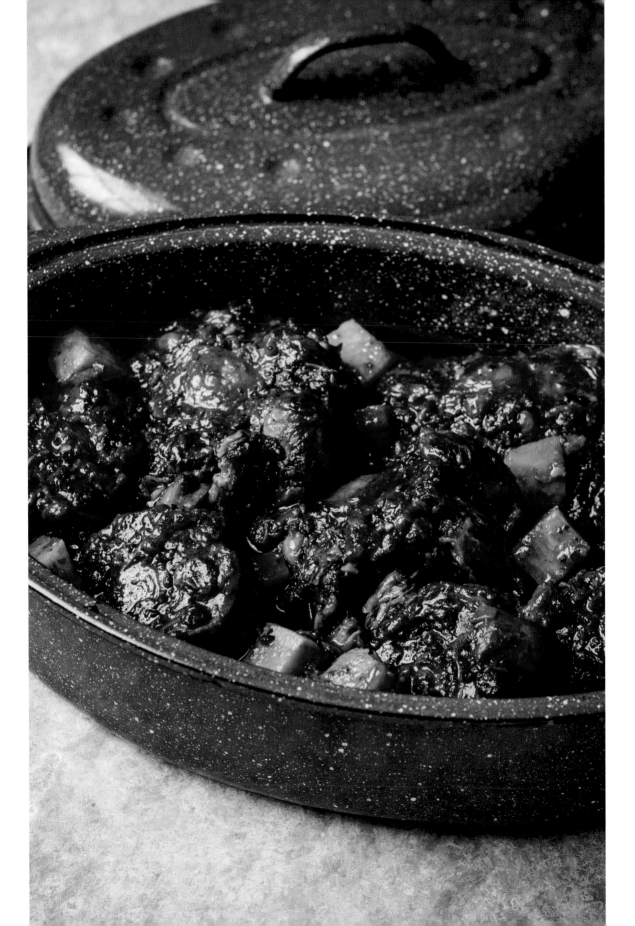

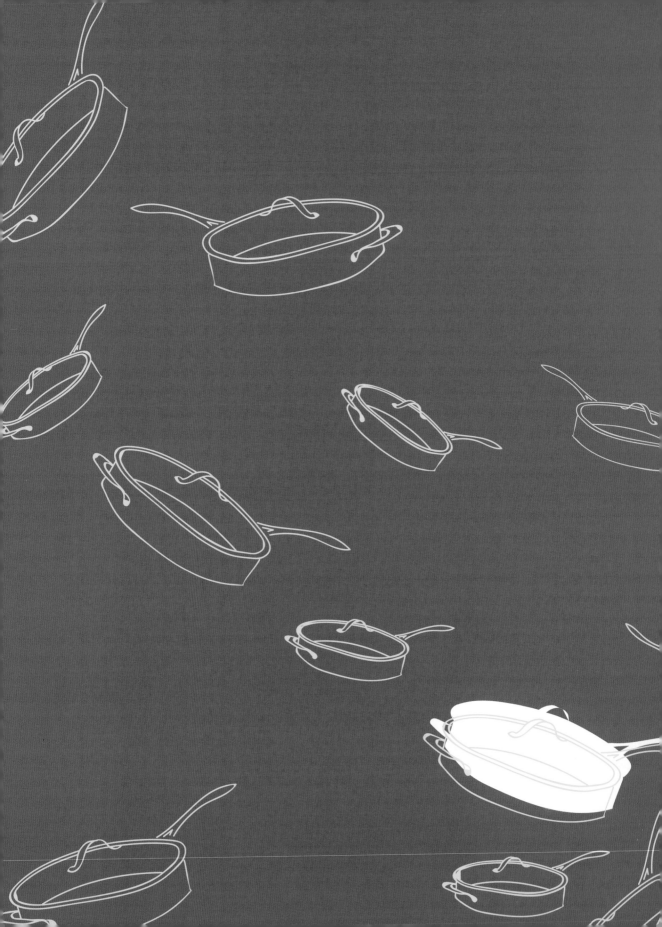

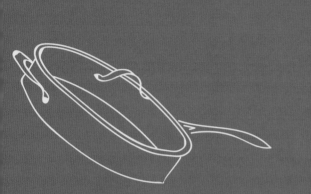

Quick
One Pot
Carbs

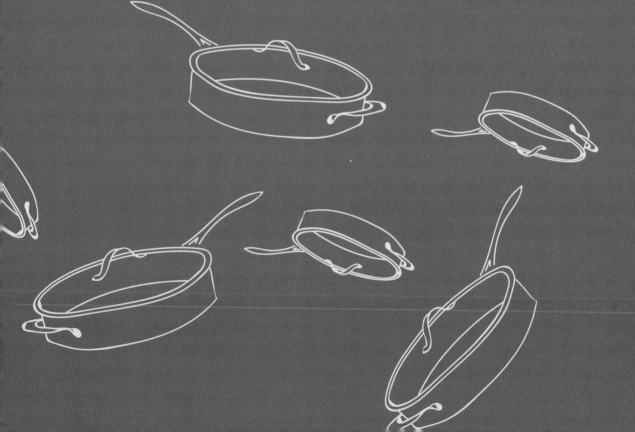

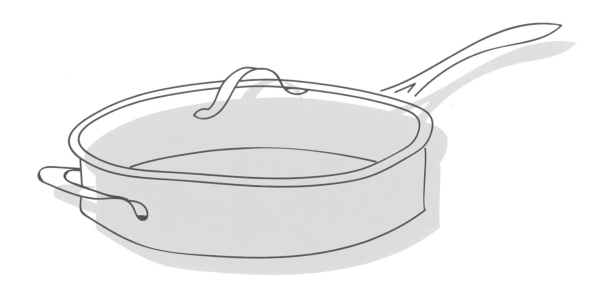

Aloo gobi 92

Egg fried rice 94

Kitchari 96

Sunblush tomato risotto 98

Mushroom and barley risotto 100

Chicken paella 102

Spring vegetable pilaf 104

Prawn and lemon risotto 106

Chicken and asparagus risotto 108

Chicken pilaf 110

Singapore noodles 112

Butternut squash and sage pasta 114

Quick pasta Bolognese 115

Spaghetti alle greens 116

Pasta e fagioli 118

Macaroni cheese 120

Tasty tuna bake 122

Aloo gobi

Although this is often served as a side dish, our version is packed with veg, so makes a good meal on its own, with some flatbread on the side. We've kept the spicing simple but there's still plenty of flavour. Everyone will gobble up this gobi.

Serves 4

3 tbsp vegetable or olive oil

1 tsp cumin seeds

½ tsp nigella seeds

½ large cauliflower, cut into florets

1 onion, finely chopped

4 garlic cloves, crushed

10g fresh root ginger, finely chopped

1 tbsp medium curry powder (shop-bought or see p.267)

400g waxy/salad potatoes, halved

2 fresh tomatoes, diced

200g frozen peas, defrosted

100g fresh spinach

salt and black pepper

To serve
chopped fresh coriander
red or green chillies, sliced
lemon wedges

Heat the oil in a large lidded sauté pan, then add the cumin and nigella seeds. When the seeds start to pop, add the cauliflower and fry briefly until it has taken on a little colour, then remove it and set aside. Add the onion and cook over a medium heat until it has softened, but don't allow it to brown. Add the garlic, ginger and curry powder and stir for a few minutes until the mixture has a paste-like consistency, then add the potatoes and stir to coat. Fry for a few minutes, then add the tomatoes and a splash of water. Season with salt and pepper.

Cover and simmer for 5 minutes, then put the cauliflower back in the pan. Turn the cauliflower over so it becomes completely coated in the sauce, then if it's looking dry, add another splash of water. Cover the pan and cook until the potatoes and cauliflower are tender, checking regularly and adding a splash more water if necessary.

Stir in the peas, then put handfuls of spinach on top and push them down into the sauce to wilt. Serve with plenty of chopped coriander and chillies and some wedges of lemon for squeezing.

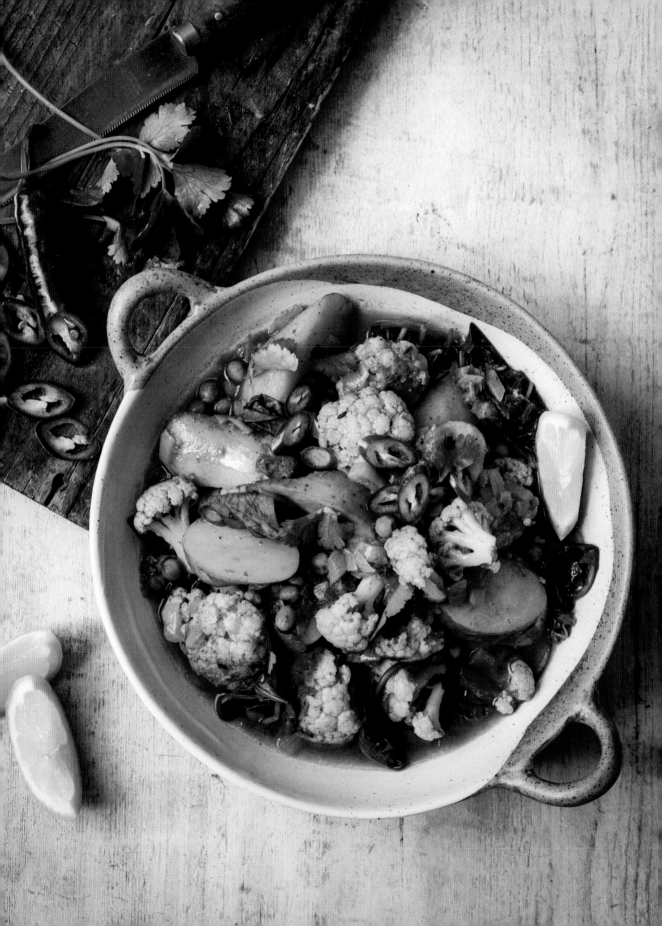

Egg fried rice

If you want a quick meal, whack it in a wok. All over Asia, the go-to one-wok wonder is egg fried rice in all its glory. Everyone loves egg fried rice and we've added chicken to our version to make it into a nourishing whole meal in a pot. It's speedy to make and good to eat.

Serves 4

2 tbsp vegetable oil

1 skinless, boneless chicken breast, cut into small dice

200g mushrooms, quartered

2 garlic cloves, finely chopped

1 red chilli, finely chopped (optional)

500g cooked and chilled long-grain rice

2 eggs, beaten

200g frozen peas, defrosted

bunch of spring onions, sliced into rounds

2 tbsp soy sauce

1 tsp sesame oil

Heat the vegetable oil in a large wok. When the air above the oil is shimmering, add the diced chicken breast and the mushrooms. Stir-fry until the chicken and mushrooms are cooked, then add the garlic and the chilli, if using. Stir-fry for a further minute, then add the rice and continue to stir-fry for a minute.

Push everything to one side of the wok, then add the beaten eggs. Stir constantly until they are lightly scrambled, then stir them into rice, together with the peas and the spring onions. Cook for a further couple of minutes, then add the soy sauce and the sesame oil. Serve at once.

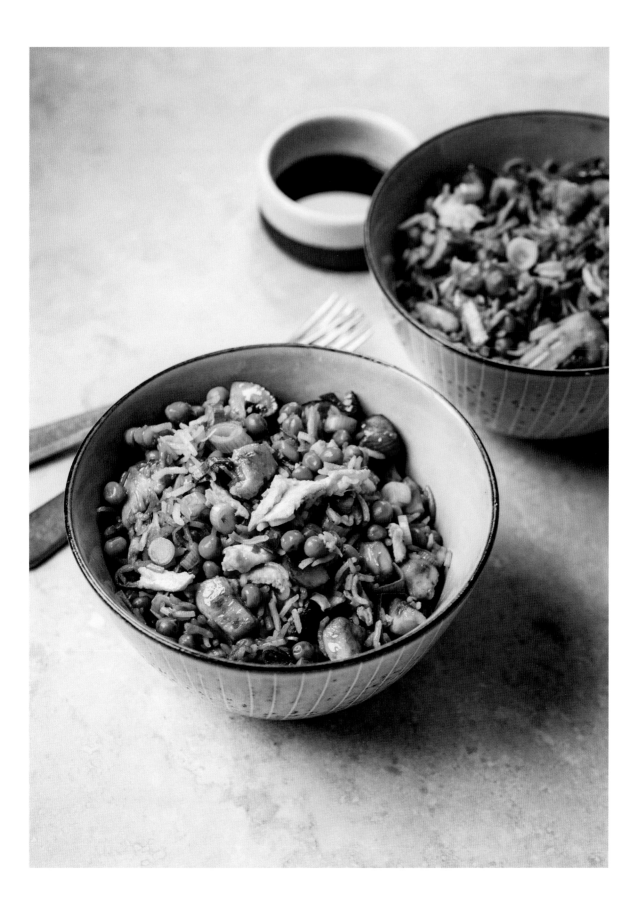

Kitchari

The word 'kitchari' means mixture in Hindi and sure enough this mildly spiced, vegan one pot dish is made with a mix of pulses and rice. It's tasty, nourishing and said to be really good for your digestion. Tastes good and does your tum good too. A perfect potful.

Serves 4

150g split yellow or red lentils

125g basmati rice

1 tbsp vegetable oil

1 tsp mustard seeds

1 tsp fennel seeds

1 onion, finely chopped

1 large carrot, very finely diced or coarsely grated

2 garlic cloves, finely chopped

15g fresh root ginger, finely chopped

1 tsp turmeric

1 tsp ground cumin

$\frac{1}{2}$ tsp ground fenugreek

1 litre vegetable stock or water

2 bay leaves

salt and black pepper

To serve
a few green chillies, finely sliced

chopped fresh coriander

lemon or lime wedges

First, thoroughly rinse the lentils and rice together, until the water runs clear.

Heat the oil in a sauté pan or a flameproof casserole dish, then add the mustard seeds and fennel seeds. When they start spitting, add the onion and cook until soft and translucent. Add the carrot, garlic, ginger and spices and continue to cook, stirring continuously, for another 2–3 minutes.

Add the rice and lentils and stir to coat them with all the spices, then add the stock or water. Season generously with salt and pepper, then add the bay leaves. Bring to the boil, then turn down the heat and cover the pan. Cook until the lentils and rice are just done – this will take 15–20 minutes. If you think the mixture is looking too dry and the lentils aren't cooked (this can happen if they are old), add more liquid.

When the lentils are cooked, remove the pan from the heat and set it aside with the lid on to steam for 5 minutes. Serve with green chillies, chopped coriander and some lemon or lime wedges for squeezing.

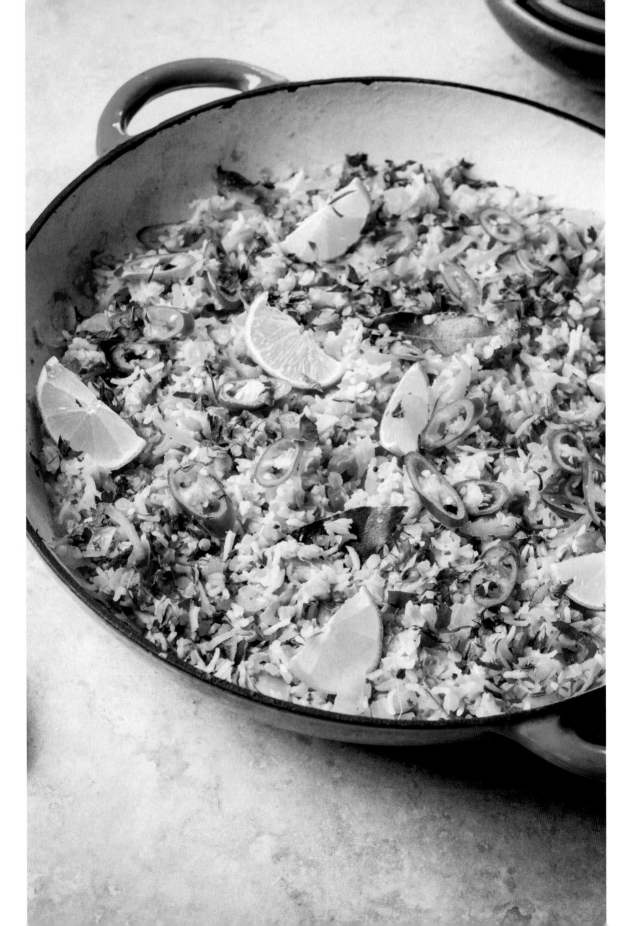

Sunblush tomato risotto

Another great veggie supper, this risotto is made with a mixture of sunblush tomatoes – available at supermarket deli counters – and cherry tomatoes, which gives a good rich sweet flavour.

Serves 4

1 tbsp olive oil

25g butter

1 onion, finely chopped

2 garlic cloves, crushed

100g sunblush tomatoes, finely chopped

2 rosemary sprigs, finely chopped

300g risotto rice

100ml white wine

1–1.2 litres vegetable stock

100g cherry tomatoes, quartered

salt and black pepper

To finish

30g butter

50g Parmesan cheese (or vegetarian alternative), grated, plus extra to serve

Heat the oil and butter in a large sauté pan or a flameproof casserole dish. When the butter is foaming, add the onion and cook gently until very soft, then turn up the heat to caramelise it around the edges. Add the garlic, sunblush tomatoes, rosemary and rice, then stir for a couple of minutes until the rice is glossy with oil and butter. Season with plenty of salt and pepper.

Add the white wine and let it boil away to nothing. Turn down the heat and start adding the stock a ladleful at a time, stirring constantly and only adding more when most of the liquid has been absorbed. When you have added at least two-thirds of the stock, add the cherry tomatoes and then continue to add the remaining stock.

When the rice is cooked to al dente and is thick enough for you to trace a clean trail along the bottom of the pan with a spoon, add the butter and Parmesan cheese and beat them into the risotto until it looks creamy. Serve with more Parmesan sprinkled over.

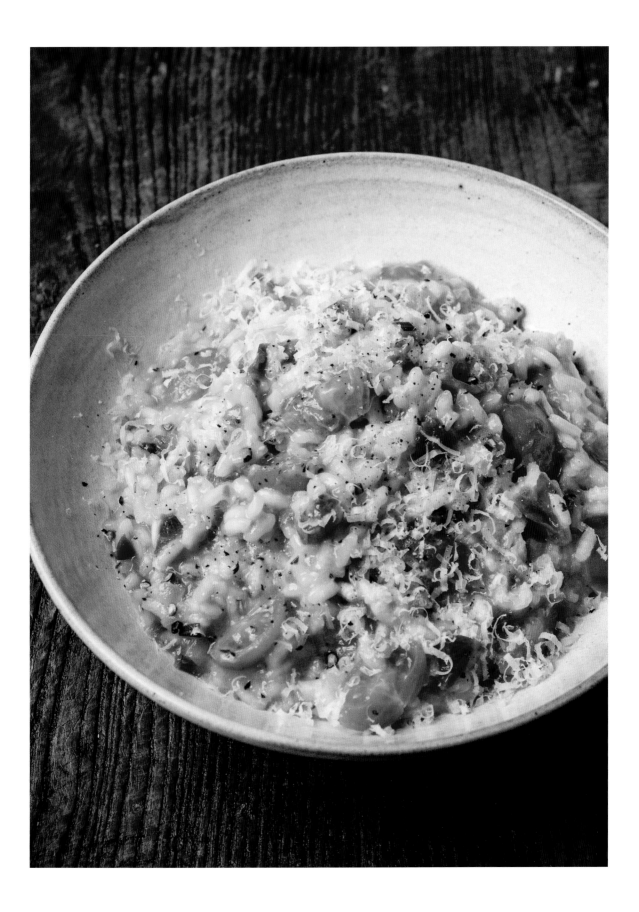

Mushroom and barley risotto

Barley is good stuff. It makes a good veggie risotto and it's higher in fibre than rice – we all know we should be eating plenty of the rough stuff. We've made the beetroot optional here but we do recommend it. Its earthy flavour goes well with the mushrooms and chard and it adds great colour to this lush, robust dish.

Serves 4

2 tbsp olive oil

25g butter

400g mushrooms, a mixture of chestnut, Portobello and white, halved or chopped if large

1 onion, finely chopped

1 bunch of chard, stems and leaves separated, shredded

10g dried mushrooms, soaked in 50ml warm water

3 garlic cloves, finely chopped

1 large thyme sprig

200g pearl barley

100ml white wine

1 litre vegetable stock

2 cooked (vac-packed) beetroots, diced (optional)

salt and black pepper

To finish

25g butter

50g Parmesan cheese (or vegetarian alternative), grated

finely chopped dill or parsley

Heat half the olive oil and half the butter in a large lidded sauté pan or a flameproof casserole dish. When the butter has melted and started to foam, add the mushrooms and cook them over a high heat until browned. Remove them and set aside.

Add the remaining oil and butter to the pan and cook the onion and chard stems over a low heat until the onion has softened and is translucent. Drain the dried mushrooms from their soaking water, reserving the water, and chop them finely. Add the mushrooms to the pan, then stir in the garlic, thyme and barley. When the barley is coated with the oil and butter and looks glossy, pour in the white wine.

Turn up the heat and cook until most of the wine has boiled off. Season generously with salt and pepper, then add the stock and the soaking liquid from the mushrooms. Bring to the boil, then turn the heat down and leave the risotto to cook, uncovered, for 20 minutes, stirring regularly.

Add the fried fresh mushrooms, the chard greens and the beetroots, if using, to the pan and stir them in. Continue to cook until the greens are tender and the barley has plumped up. The barley should have a texture similar to risotto – you should be able to see a clear path when you draw your wooden spoon along the base of the pan. Beat in the butter and Parmesan, check the seasoning, then serve with chopped dill or parsley.

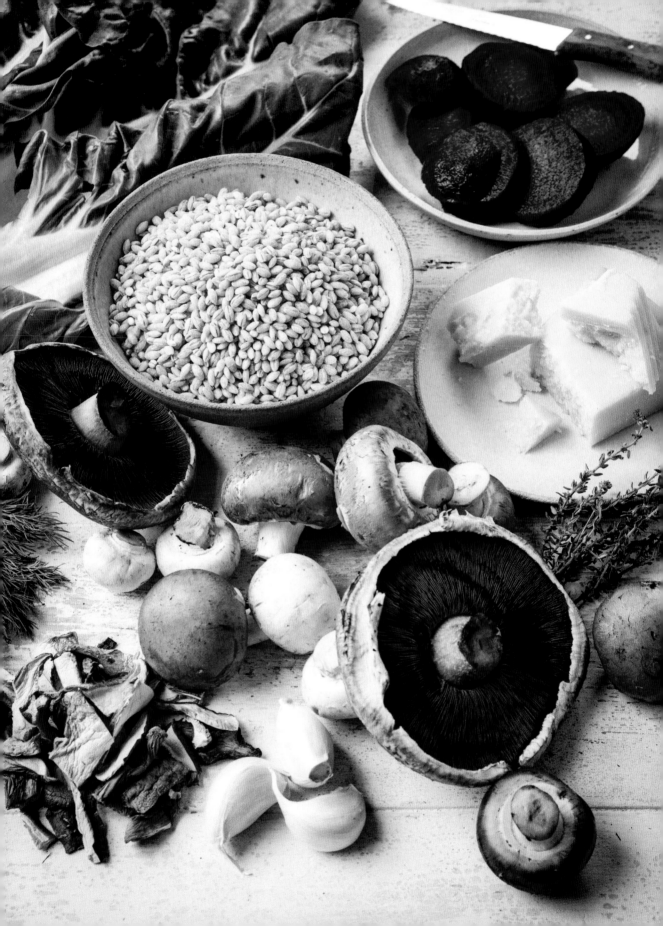

Chicken paella

It doesn't take long to bang the chicken into a marinade of olive oil, lemon and oregano and it really does make a difference to the flavour of this dish. This isn't a completely authentic paella but it's easy to make and tastes epic. Get your flamenco gear on and dig in.

Serves 6

6 skinless, boneless chicken thighs, diced

3 tbsp olive oil

zest and juice of 1 lemon

1 tsp dried oregano

1 large onion, finely chopped

4 garlic cloves, finely chopped

1 tsp sweet paprika

1 large rosemary sprig, finely chopped

2 tomatoes, peeled and finely chopped

100ml white wine

1 tsp saffron strands, soaked in 2 tbsp warm water

up to 1.2 litres chicken or vegetable stock

500g paella rice

6 chargrilled artichokes, halved (from a jar or the deli counter)

150g green beans, trimmed

salt and black pepper

To serve
lemon wedges

Toss the diced chicken in a tablespoon of the oil, the lemon zest and juice and the oregano, then season well with salt and pepper. Set the chicken aside to marinate while you start the paella.

Heat the remaining oil in a large paella pan or a frying pan, then add the onion. Cook over a medium to low heat until the onion is soft and translucent. Turn up the heat, drain the chicken from the marinade and add it to the pan. Cook the chicken until it is lightly coloured on all sides, then add the garlic, paprika, rosemary and tomatoes. Stir to coat the chicken and cook until the moisture from the tomatoes has evaporated.

Pour in the white wine and allow it to bubble up for a minute or so, then add the saffron strands and the stock. Season with salt and pepper, then bring to the boil. Sprinkle in the rice, spacing it out as evenly as possible and making sure the chicken is evenly distributed around the pan. This is important, as this is the only time you should stir the paella.

Arrange the artichokes and green beans over the rice and let them sink into the stock. Bring to the boil and cook for 5 minutes. Turn down the heat and leave the rice to simmer gently until it is cooked through. This should take 12–15 minutes. If you think the paella is getting too dry before the rice is completely cooked through, add another ladleful of stock or water. The rice should be al dente when it is cooked.

Take the pan off the heat, then cover the paella with a lid or preferably a damp tea towel and leave it to stand for 10 minutes to steam in its own heat. Serve with lemon wedges for squeezing over.

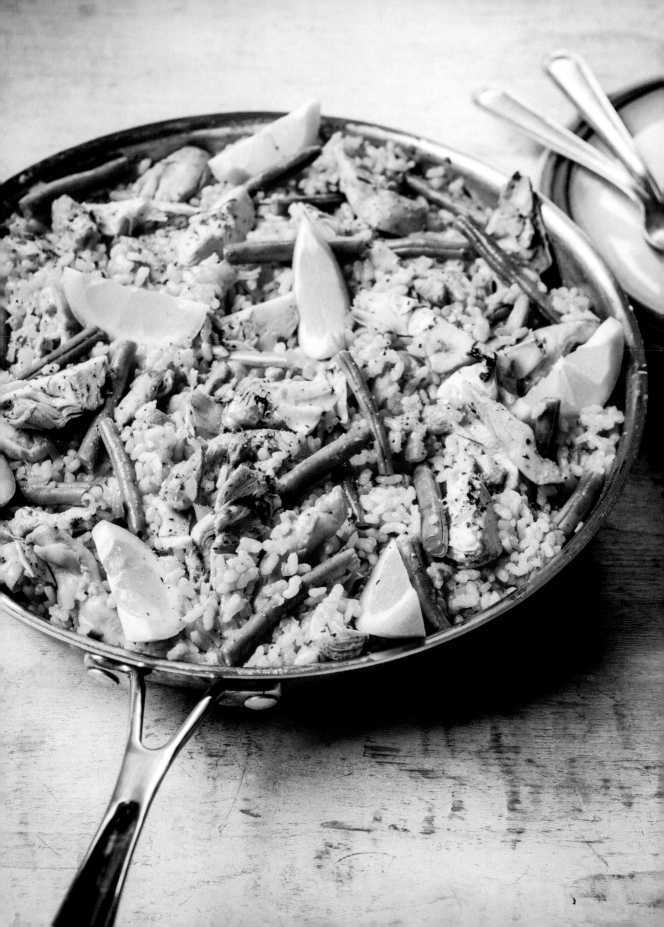

Spring vegetable pilaf

This idea came from a Turkish broad bean and dill pilaf we cooked way back, and we've expanded it from a side dish to a beautiful main meal. There's loads of veg in this dish and you can vary them if you like – use spinach or kale instead of chard, for instance. And if you want to make this a vegan meal, just use an extra tablespoon of oil instead of the butter. If peeling the skins off the broad beans seems like too much of a faff, don't bother, but they do look – and taste – better. Get someone else to help.

Serves 4

2 tbsp olive oil

15g butter

1 onion, finely chopped

small bunch of chard, stems and leaves separated and shredded

1 large courgette, finely chopped

300–400g frozen broad beans (see method)

300g basmati rice

½ tsp allspice

¼ tsp cinnamon

pinch of saffron

bunch of asparagus tips, thinly sliced on the diagonal

100g frozen peas

large bunch of dill, finely chopped

small bunch of mint, leaves only, chopped

zest of 1 lime

Salt

To serve
lime wedges

Greek yoghurt

Heat the oil and butter in a large flameproof casserole dish. When the butter has melted, add the onion, chard stems and courgette. Cook over a gentle heat until the onion is soft and translucent.

While the onion is cooking, prepare the broad beans. Pour a kettle of boiling water over them, then drain and slip off the grey outer skins. You should end up with about 300g of beans, so if you don't want to peel your broad beans, just use this amount instead.

Cover the rice in cold water and swill it around, until the water turns cloudy. Strain and repeat until the water runs clear.

When the onion is cooked, add the spices to the pan, then pour in 500ml of water and add plenty of salt. Bring to the boil, then add the rice, followed by the chard greens. Give everything a quick stir, then add the asparagus, broad beans and peas. Cover and leave to cook for 15 minutes. Check – if the rice is still very firm, leave for another 3–4 minutes, then remove the pan from the heat and leave to stand for at least another 10 minutes to steam.

Stir through the dill and mint leaves. Serve immediately, with wedges of lime and plenty of yoghurt.

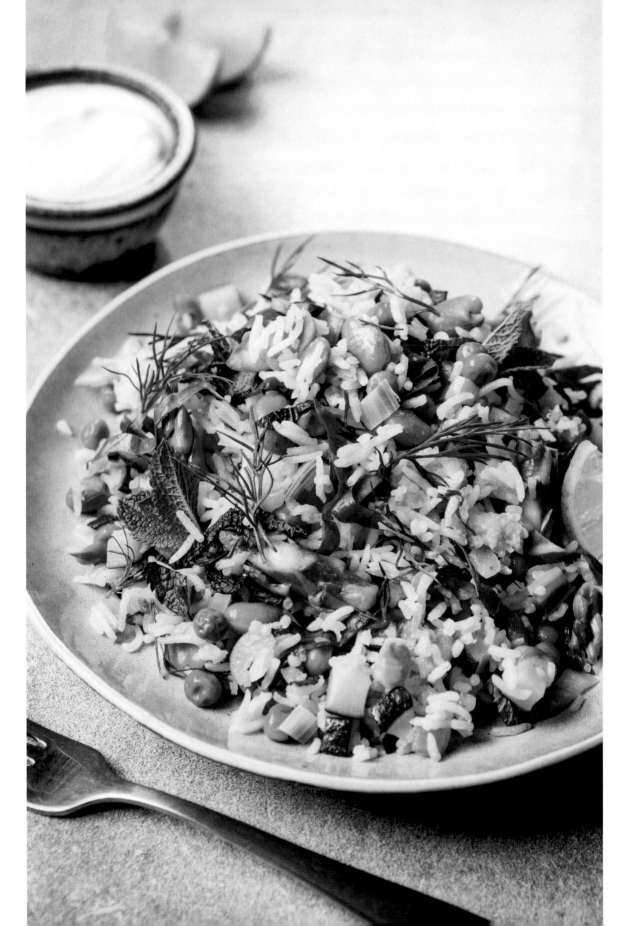

Prawn and lemon risotto

Prawns and rice are one of our favourite combos and this is a really zesty fresh risotto. We know there's a bit of stirring to do, but just put some music on, relax and enjoy. This is proper comfort food. Pavarotti would be proud of us.

Serves 4

1 tbsp olive oil
400g raw shelled prawns
50g butter
1 onion, finely chopped
1 courgette, finely diced
2 garlic cloves, finely chopped
300g risotto rice
zest of 1 lemon
100ml white wine
1.2 litres fish, vegetable or
  chicken stock
25g Parmesan cheese, grated
salt and black pepper

To serve
basil leaves
Parmesan cheese, grated

Heat the oil in a flameproof casserole dish or a sauté pan. Add the prawns in a single layer and sear them on both sides over a high heat, then remove them from the pan. Turn down the heat and add half the butter. When it has melted and started to foam, add the onion and courgette. Sauté until the onion is soft and translucent and the courgette is soft around the edges. Add the garlic and stir for a minute or so, then stir in the rice.

When the rice is glossy and coated with butter, stir in the lemon zest and turn up the heat. Add the wine and bring it to the boil. When the wine has reduced down to almost nothing, season with salt and pepper, then start adding the stock a ladleful at a time, stirring in between each addition, until most of the liquid has been absorbed by the rice. When the rice starts to look plump and you can make a clear path when you pull your spoon through it, the risotto should be ready – al dente and creamy. Taste for seasoning, then beat in the remaining butter and the Parmesan.

Put the prawns back in the pan with any liquid they might have given out while resting. Warm them through, then take the pan off the heat and garnish the risotto with a few basil leaves. Serve with more Parmesan.

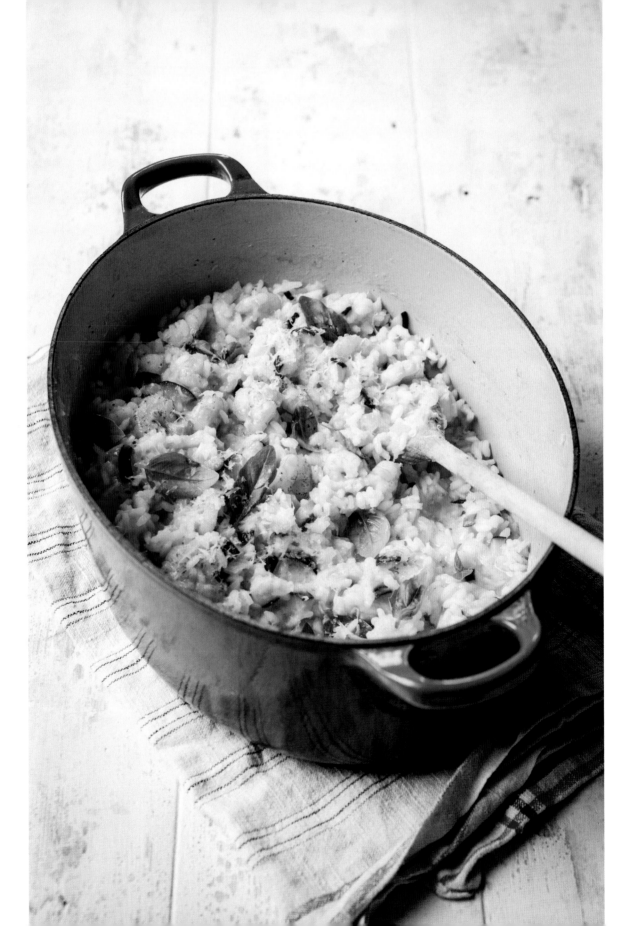

Chicken and asparagus risotto

We both love asparagus but it is a bit pricey, so we like to use it in dishes like risotto where you don't need loads but it provides great flavour. Asparagus goes really well with chicken too.

Serves 4

200g long asparagus stems

1 tbsp olive oil

4 skinless, boneless chicken thighs, diced

50g butter

1 large onion, finely chopped

2 small courgettes, sliced into thin rounds

2 garlic cloves, finely chopped

1 strip of pared lemon zest

300g risotto rice

100ml white wine

about 1.25 litres chicken stock

50g Parmesan cheese, grated, plus extra to serve

salt and black pepper

First prepare the asparagus. Bend each stem and snap off the woody ends where they break naturally. Discard the woody ends or save them to use in soup. Cut the tips from the stems and slice the stems into rounds.

Heat the oil in a large sauté pan or a flameproof casserole dish. Add the asparagus tips and cook them over a high heat until they're lightly browned and tender to the point of a knife. Remove them from the pan. Add the diced chicken and fry until browned and just cooked through. Remove and set aside.

Add half the butter to the pan. When it has melted and started to foam, add the onion and cook over a medium heat for 5 minutes. Add the asparagus stems and courgette rounds and continue to cook until the onion is soft and translucent, then stir in the garlic and lemon zest. Cook for another 2 minutes.

Add the risotto rice and stir so the grains are glossy and well coated in the buttery juices. Season with salt and pepper. Turn up the heat and pour in the wine. Allow it to bubble up fiercely for a minute or so until most of it has boiled off, then turn down the heat. Add a ladleful of the stock and stir continuously until most of it has evaporated or been absorbed by the rice, then repeat until all the stock is incorporated. The rice should be al dente with a creamy sauce around it.

Add the remaining butter and the Parmesan and beat them in thoroughly – this will give the risotto a creamy texture. Stir in the cooked chicken and the asparagus, then cover the pan and leave for a couple of minutes, just to warm them through. Serve immediately with more Parmesan cheese grated over the top.

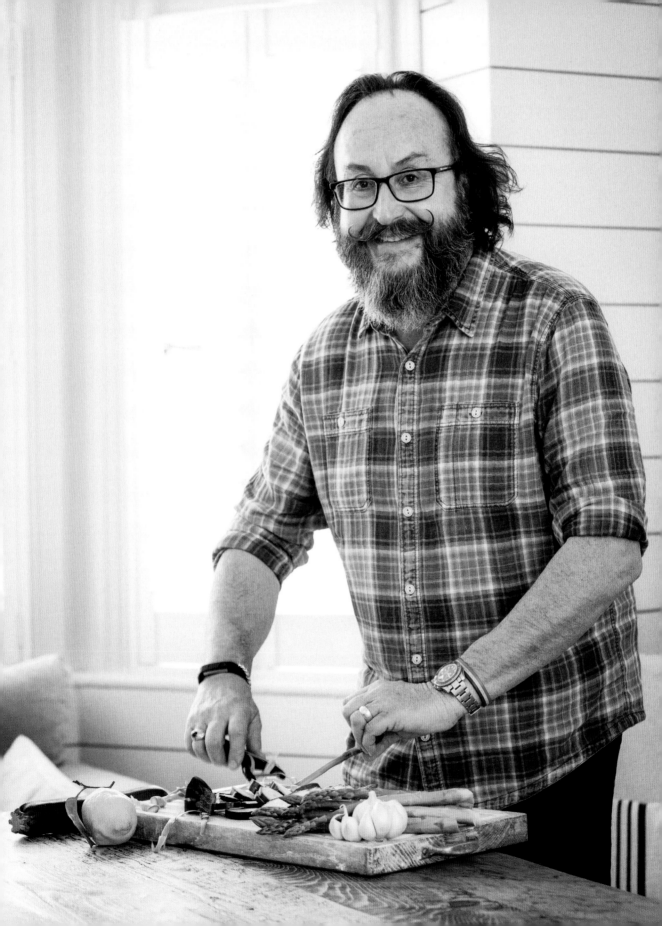

Chicken pilaf

If you don't like stirring, make a pilaf instead of a risotto. The dish is drier, not creamy, but still full of flavour. We wanted to find a way of making sure this pilaf was nice and juicy, so we came up with the idea of adding pomegranate seeds. They look good and you get a burst of delicious juice with every mouthful.

Serves 4

200ml yoghurt

pinch of saffron

zest and juice of ½ lime

6 skinless, boneless chicken
  thighs, diced

400g basmati rice

1 tbsp olive oil

15g butter

1 onion, finely chopped

25g pistachios, roughly
  chopped

15g fresh root ginger, finely
  chopped

2 garlic cloves, finely chopped

2 tsp ground coriander

1 tsp ground cardamom

½ tsp cinnamon

½ tsp allspice

¼ tsp mace or nutmeg

2 bay leaves

50g raisins (green or yellow
  if possible)

800ml chicken stock

salt and black pepper

To serve
seeds from half a large
pomegranate

chopped parsley

chopped fresh coriander

Mix the yoghurt with the saffron and the lime zest and juice. Season the chicken with salt and pepper, then add it to the yoghurt. Stir to coat the chicken, then leave it to marinate for an hour if you have time.

Cover the rice in cold water and swill it around, until the water turns cloudy. Strain and repeat until the water runs clear.

Heat the oil and butter in a large flameproof casserole dish. Add the onion and cook gently until it's soft and translucent, then add the pistachios. Cook until the pistachios start to brown, then add the ginger, garlic, spices, bay leaves and raisins. Stir until everything is well combined, then add the chicken. Cook it over a high heat for 2–3 minutes, stirring so it becomes coated with all the spices. Add the drained rice and do the same.

Add a little stock to the casserole dish to deglaze it, making sure you give the base a good scrape, then pour in the rest of the stock. Season with salt and pepper, bring to the boil, then turn down the heat and cover the pan. Cook for 15 minutes until all the liquid has been absorbed, then remove the pan from the heat and leave to stand, covered, for another 10 minutes. The rice will continue to steam during this time and will become fluffier.

Garnish the pilaf with the pomegranate seeds and the herbs and serve.

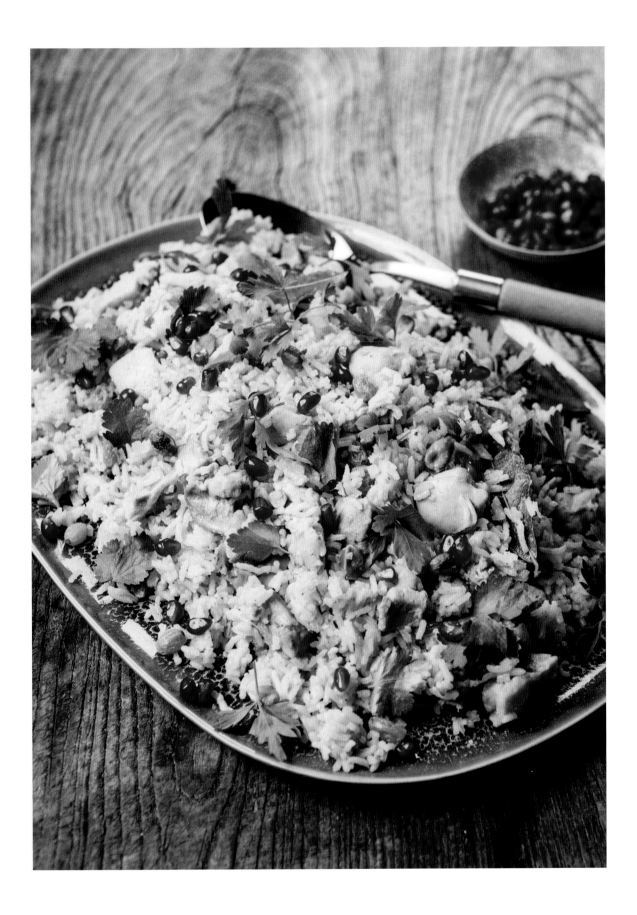

Singapore noodles

This is Dave's go-to dish in Chinese restaurants. It is traditionally made with rice vermicelli, but if you fancy a bit of a chow mein vibe, use egg noodles. You might be surprised to know that no one knows about this dish in Singapore. We think it was invented in Hong Kong but whatever the story, it's great to eat. This is a quick version and makes a cracking good supper. A guilty pleasure.

Serves 4

200g rice or egg vermicelli

2 tbsp vegetable oil

1 onion, sliced into thin wedges

1 carrot, cut into matchsticks

1 red pepper, thinly sliced

2 garlic cloves, finely chopped

10g fresh root ginger, finely chopped

200g pork tenderloin, finely sliced

225g can of bamboo shoots, drained

25g frozen peas, defrosted

1 tsp Chinese 5-spice powder

2 tsp mild curry powder

2 tbsp light soy sauce

1 tbsp rice wine

1 tbsp rice wine vinegar

75g cooked shelled prawns

To garnish

1 tsp sesame oil

2 spring onions, shredded

1 green or red chilli, finely sliced (optional)

chopped fresh coriander

Cover the noodles with freshly boiled water and leave them to stand for a minute. Drain and set aside until you are ready for them.

Heat the oil in a large wok. Add the onion, carrot and red pepper and stir-fry over a high heat until they're starting to brown. Add the garlic, ginger and pork and continue to stir-fry until the pork is coloured on all sides. Tip in the bamboo shoots, peas, spices, soy sauce, rice wine and rice wine vinegar, then add the noodles and stir thoroughly to combine. Leave to cook for a couple of minutes until hot.

Stir in the prawns and heat them through, then serve with a drizzle of sesame oil and sprinkled with the spring onions, chilli, if using, and coriander.

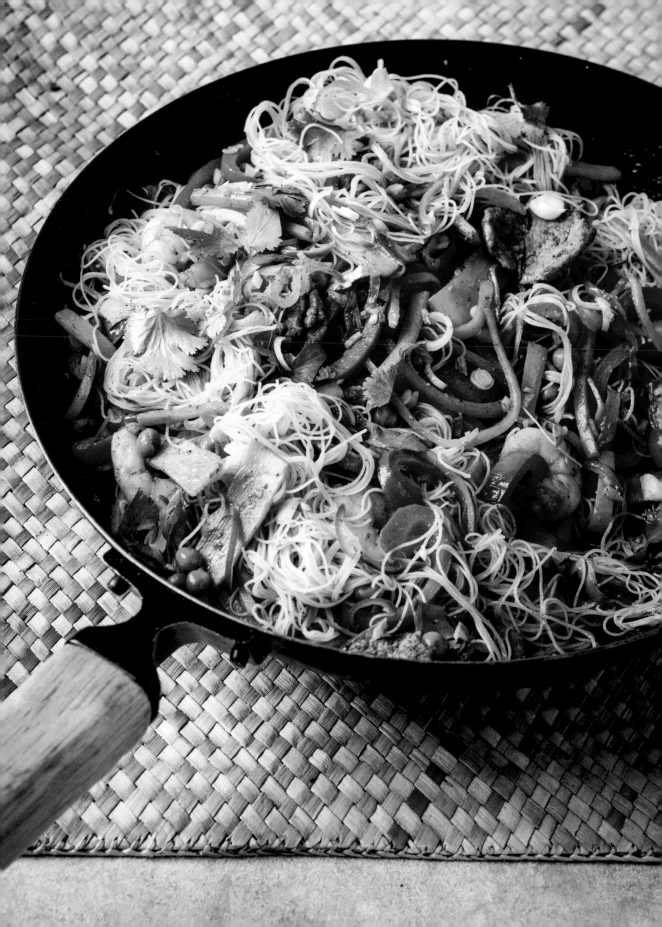

Butternut squash and sage pasta

Pasta is the go-to quick supper in many homes, including ours and this one-pan absorption method makes it even quicker and easier. The pasta and sauce is all cooked together so increasing the flavour and halving the washing up! You could add a couple of cut-up sausages with the leeks and squash if you like.

Serves 4

2 tbsp olive oil

15g butter

2 leeks, cut into rounds

500g butternut squash, peeled and diced

2 garlic cloves, finely chopped

1 tsp rubbed sage

100ml white wine

500g short pasta, such as penne

1.5 litres vegetable or chicken stock

100ml double cream

a few rasps of nutmeg

salt and black pepper

To serve

Parmesan cheese (or vegetarian alternative), grated

Heat the olive oil and butter in a large flameproof casserole dish or a saucepan. Add the leeks and butternut squash and cook for 5 minutes over a medium heat, stirring regularly. Add the garlic, sage and white wine and bring to the boil. Cover the pan and leave the veg to simmer for a further 5 minutes, by which time the leeks should be tender to the point of a knife.

Stir in the pasta and season with salt and pepper, then pour in the stock. Bring to the boil, then turn down the heat, cover and leave to simmer, stirring regularly. When the pasta has cooked and most of the liquid has been absorbed, remove the pan from the heat and leave to stand for 5 minutes. Pour in the cream and grate in the nutmeg, then stir to combine.

Serve with plenty of Parmesan cheese.

Quick pasta Bolognese

Another speedy pasta supper, this time with a very simple Bolognese sauce. Yum! The cheese added at the end brings a richness to the sauce. A bit clever this one and none of the lovely flavours are lost.

Serves 4

1 onion, roughly chopped

1 carrot, roughly chopped

2 celery sticks, roughly chopped

3 tbsp olive oil

400g minced beef

3 garlic cloves, finely chopped

2 tbsp tomato purée

1 tsp dried oregano

2 bay leaves

250ml red wine

500g short pasta, such as penne

1.5 litres beef stock

100g Cheddar cheese, grated

salt and black pepper

To serve
Parmesan cheese, grated

a few basil leaves

Put the onion, carrot and celery into a food processor. Pulse until the vegetables are very finely chopped – almost to, but not quite, a purée.

Heat the olive oil in a large flameproof casserole dish or a saucepan. Add the blitzed vegetables and cook over a medium heat until they're softened and starting to take on some colour. Turn up the heat, add the beef and cook until it is browned on all sides. Add the garlic and continue to cook for another 2 minutes.

Stir in the tomato purée and cook for another 2–3 minutes, stirring constantly, then add the herbs and red wine. Bring to the boil and cook until the wine has reduced to almost nothing. Season with salt and pepper.

Stir in the pasta, then cover with the stock. Bring to the boil, then turn the heat down to a simmer and cover the pan. Leave to cook for 20 minutes, stirring gently every so often to make sure the pasta cooks evenly.

When the pasta is cooked through, remove the lid and leave to simmer for a few minutes longer to make sure the sauce is well reduced. Stir in the Cheddar cheese, then serve, sprinkled with Parmesan and basil leaves.

Spaghetti alle greens

This is a clever dish, though we say it ourselves. The pasta and veg are all cooked together, then tossed with a little of the cooking liquid, some oil, seasonings and lemon. The result is awesome and it's so quick and easy. Fresh and genius.

Serves 4

400g spaghetti or linguini

150g broad beans (frozen are fine)

150g spinach or rocket

1 tbsp olive oil

1 large courgette, coarsely grated and squeezed of excess liquid

1 garlic clove, crushed

zest of 1 lemon

75g Parmesan cheese (or vegetarian alternative), grated

handful of basil leaves, shredded

salt and black pepper

Heat a large pan of water. When it is at a rolling boil, add plenty of salt and the pasta. Check the cooking instructions on the pasta and make a note of the cooking time.

When the pasta is 3 minutes away from being ready, add the broad beans – no need to remove the skins unless you feel like it. After a further 2 minutes, add the spinach or rocket. When the greens have wilted down and the pasta is al dente, reserve a couple of ladlefuls of the cooking liquid and drain the pasta thoroughly.

Tip the pasta back into the pan and add the olive oil. Toss lightly, add the courgette, garlic, lemon zest and Parmesan, then season with more salt and plenty of black pepper. Stir in some of the reserved cooking liquid – you don't want a liquid sauce, so add just enough to stop the pasta looking claggy or dry. Stir in the basil and serve immediately.

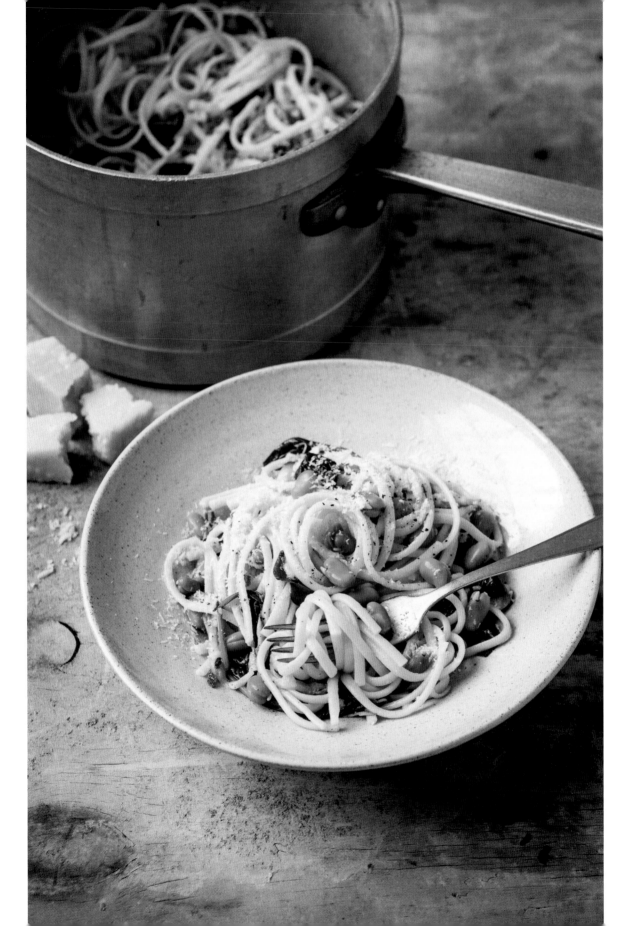

Pasta e fagioli

Pasta and beans – this classic Italian dish is one of our favourites. It's hearty and filling, and our version is also packed with vegetables so it's a great way of enjoying your five a day! Dead simple to make too.

Serves 4

2 tbsp olive oil

100g smoked bacon lardons

1 large onion, roughly diced

200g butternut squash, diced

3 celery sticks, diced

100g chard, stems and leaves separated, shredded

3 garlic cloves, finely chopped

3 rosemary sprigs

Parmesan rind (optional)

1 litre vegetable or chicken stock

150g short pasta, such as fusilli

2 x 400g cans of borlotti beans, drained

4 tomatoes, roughly chopped

salt and black pepper

To serve
Parmesan cheese, grated
finely chopped parsley

Heat the oil in a large flameproof casserole dish or a saucepan. Add the bacon, onion, squash, celery and the chard stems and cook over a medium heat for 10–15 minutes, until the veg are starting to soften.

Add the garlic, rosemary and Parmesan rind, if using, and pour in the stock. Season with salt and pepper, then bring to the boil. Cover and simmer for 15 minutes until the vegetables are al dente, then add the pasta and beans. Cook for 5 minutes, then add the shredded chard leaves and the tomatoes. Simmer until the pasta is just done and the vegetables are tender.

Serve sprinkled with grated Parmesan and lots of chopped parsley.

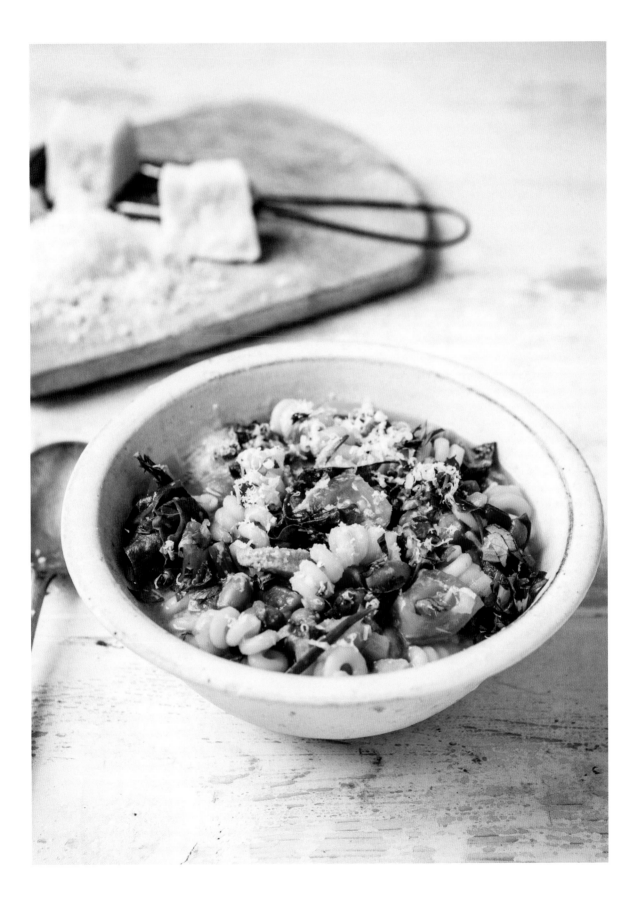

Macaroni cheese

Yes, mac 'n' cheese all in one pot! No faffing about making a cheese sauce. The dish works because the starch from the pasta is released and combines with the milk and water to thicken the sauce. Magic!

Serves 4

1 tbsp olive oil

15g butter

1 onion, finely chopped

100g smoked bacon, diced

2 garlic cloves, finely chopped

1 tsp dried thyme

500g macaroni (preferably elbow macaroni)

750ml whole milk

2 tbsp wholegrain mustard

150g cherry tomatoes, halved

200g mature Cheddar cheese, grated

salt and black pepper

Heat the olive oil and butter in a large flameproof casserole dish. Add the onion and bacon and cook until the onion is soft and translucent. Turn up the heat, then continue to cook until the bacon is crisp and has rendered out much of its fat. Don't worry if the onion browns too, it will add to the flavour.

Stir in the garlic and thyme and continue to cook for 2 minutes, then add the macaroni. Pour in the milk and 750ml of water, then stir in the mustard. Season well with salt and pepper. Bring to the boil, then turn down the heat and leave everything to simmer, uncovered, for 8–10 minutes or until the macaroni is cooked and most of the liquid has been absorbed. You want the texture quite loose, so add a little more water or milk if necessary. Preheat your grill to its highest setting.

Add the cherry tomatoes and 150g of the cheese and stir until the cheese has melted, then leave the pan over a low heat for a further 5 minutes, just to allow the tomatoes to soften. Sprinkle over the remaining cheese and put the dish under the grill until the cheese has melted and browned.

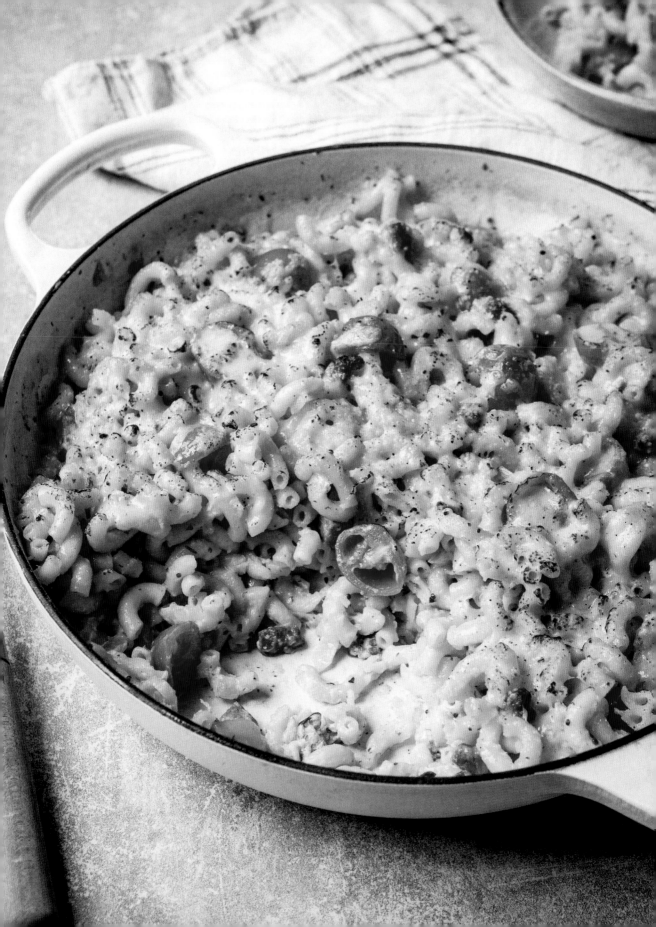

Tasty tuna bake

Everyone loves a tuna bake for supper and this version is cooked all in one. There's no boiling the pasta in a separate pan, as it cooks by the absorption method. We've added gutsy flavours such as capers, olives and chilli to make this a real crowd pleaser.

Serves 4

2 tbsp olive oil

1 onion, finely chopped

2 garlic cloves, finely chopped

2 cans of tuna in spring water, drained

400g can of chopped tomatoes

25g capers, roughly chopped

25g black olives, roughly chopped

1 tsp lemon zest

leaves from a thyme sprig

½ tsp chilli flakes (optional)

400g short pasta, such as fusilli or penne

75g Cheddar cheese, grated

salt and black pepper

Heat the olive oil in a large flameproof casserole dish with a lid and add the onion. Cook until the onion is very soft and translucent, then add the garlic. Cook for another couple of minutes, then add the tuna, tomatoes, capers, olives and lemon zest. Sprinkle in the thyme and the chilli flakes, if using. Stir everything together until well combined, then add the pasta. Season with salt and pepper, then stir again, making sure all the pasta is completely coated with the sauce.

Pour in enough water to just cover the pasta and bring to the boil. Turn down the heat to a simmer and cover the pan. Cook until the pasta is al dente and has absorbed most of the water – stir every now and again to make sure the pasta isn't sticking to the base of the dish. Heat your grill to its highest setting.

The pasta should be cooked in about 15 minutes, but start checking a few minutes before as pasta varies so much. Sprinkle with cheese and put the dish, uncovered, under the hot grill until bubbling and brown. Serve at once.

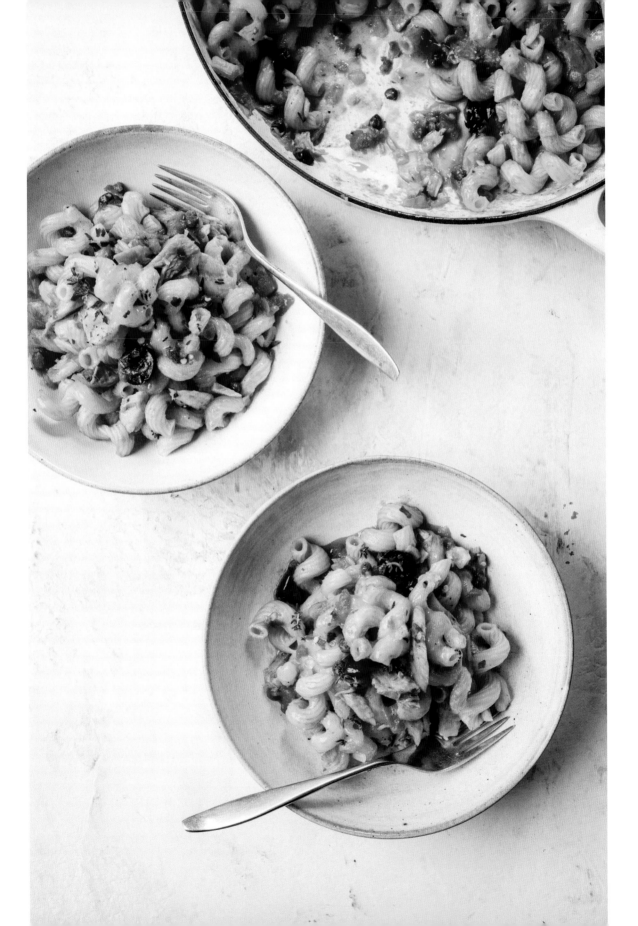

Tarts and Tray Bakes

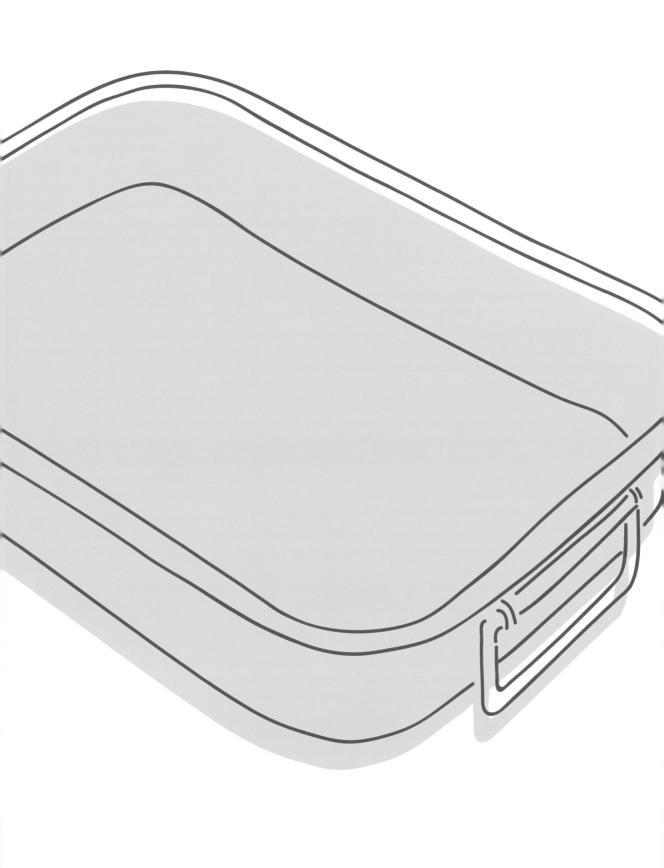

Showstopper quiche

This is more than your average quiche, with lots of veg as well as eggs and cheese. Quiches can be a bit fiddly, but the filling ingredients for this one don't have to be precooked, which makes for an easy life. Everything can be put straight into the pastry case and baked together. Use bought pastry if you like or try our recipe on page 273 – make double the quantity and stash some in the freezer for another time.

Serves 4

400g shortcrust pastry (shop-bought or see p. 273)

plain flour, for rolling

1 tbsp wholegrain mustard

300g frozen spinach, defrosted

50g rocket, roughly chopped

a few tarragon sprigs, roughly chopped

75g Cheddar or Gruyère cheese, grated

4 spring onions, finely sliced

4 eggs

200ml crème fraiche

100ml double cream

100g cherry tomatoes, halved

salt and black pepper

Preheat the oven to 200°C/Fan 180°C/Gas 6. Roll out the pastry on a floured work surface and use it to line a 25cm round flan dish. Prick the pastry all over with a fork, then cover it with greaseproof paper and fill with baking beans. Bake in the oven for 15 minutes, then remove the paper and beans and cook the pastry for another 5 minutes until the base is set and lightly coloured. Reduce the oven temperature to 180°C/Fan 160°C/Gas 4. Allow the pastry case to cool.

Spread the mustard over the base of the pastry. Squeeze out the liquid from the frozen spinach, and chop roughly. Mix it with the rocket and tarragon and season with salt and pepper, then stir in half the cheese. Arrange this mixture over the mustard, then sprinkle over the spring onions. Whisk the eggs with the crème fraiche and double cream and season with salt and pepper, then pour this over the greens. Top with the remaining cheese and the cherry tomatoes.

Bake the quiche in the oven for 30–35 minutes. The top will puff up, but will drop back down again once the tart cools. Serve warm or at room temperature.

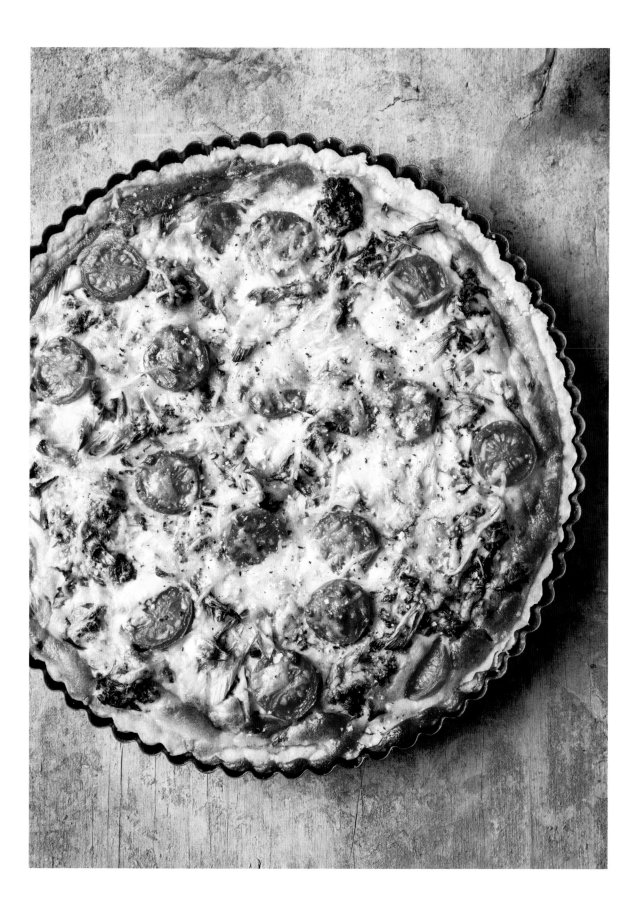

Mediterranean tart

You've got to love ready-rolled puff pastry which makes preparing open tarts so quick and easy. This recipe is a real winner and so tasty. You could also top it with some grilled Mediterranean vegetables, such as peppers and aubergines, which you can buy at the deli counter.

Serves 4

1 x 320g ready-rolled puff pastry sheet

2 tbsp red pesto (shop-bought or see p.272)

1 tbsp olive oil

1 small courgette, sliced into thin ribbons

100g cherry tomatoes, halved

a few black olives, pitted

100g block of mozzarella

a few fresh oregano sprigs

1 egg, beaten

salt and black pepper

Preheat the oven to 200°C/Fan 180°C/Gas 6. Unroll the puff pastry on to a large baking tray and score a 2cm border all the way round.

Spread the pesto over the pastry within the scored border. Put the oil in a bowl, add the courgette strips and toss to coat them in oil, then drape the strips over the pesto. Arrange the cherry tomatoes and olives around the courgettes, then pull the mozzarella into strips and add them too. Sprinkle with fresh oregano leaves.

Brush the edges of the puff pastry with beaten egg and sprinkle the whole tart with salt and pepper. Bake in the oven for 25 minutes until the pastry has puffed up and browned. Cut into slices to serve.

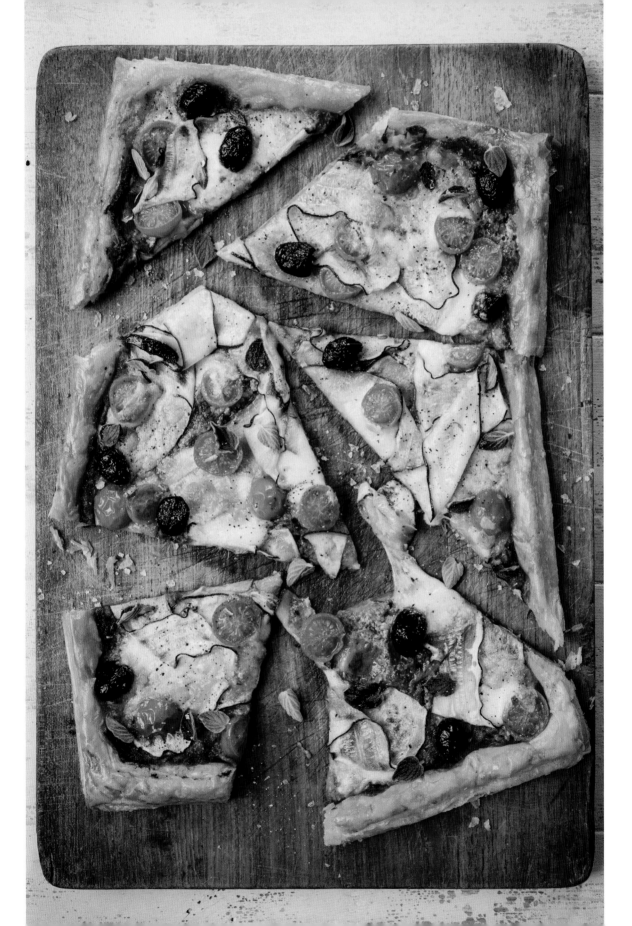

Parma ham, peach and goats' cheese tart

Dead easy this and so good. We thought of adding honey in case the peaches or nectarines were a bit sharp but actually we like it anyway and it goes really well with the goats' cheese. This is really quick to prepare, then just shove it in the oven and you have a fab lunch.

Makes 4

1 x 320g ready-rolled puff pastry sheet

2 ripe peaches or nectarines

150g goats' cheese log, sliced

80–100g pack of Parma ham

1 tbsp olive oil

1–2 tsp runny honey (optional)

1 egg, beaten

a few basil leaves

handful of rocket leaves

salt and black pepper

Preheat the oven to 200°C/Fan 180°C/Gas 6. Unroll the puff pastry on to a large baking tray. Score a 2cm border all the way round.

Cut the peaches or nectarines into wedges and arrange them over the pastry, making sure they stay within the scored lines. Add the slices of cheese, then drape over the slices of Parma ham. Brush the peaches with olive oil and the honey, if using, then brush the border of the puff pastry with the beaten egg. Season with salt and pepper.

Bake in the oven for 20–25 minutes until the pastry has puffed up, particularly around the edges, and everything is well browned. Sprinkle over the basil and the rocket leaves and serve immediately.

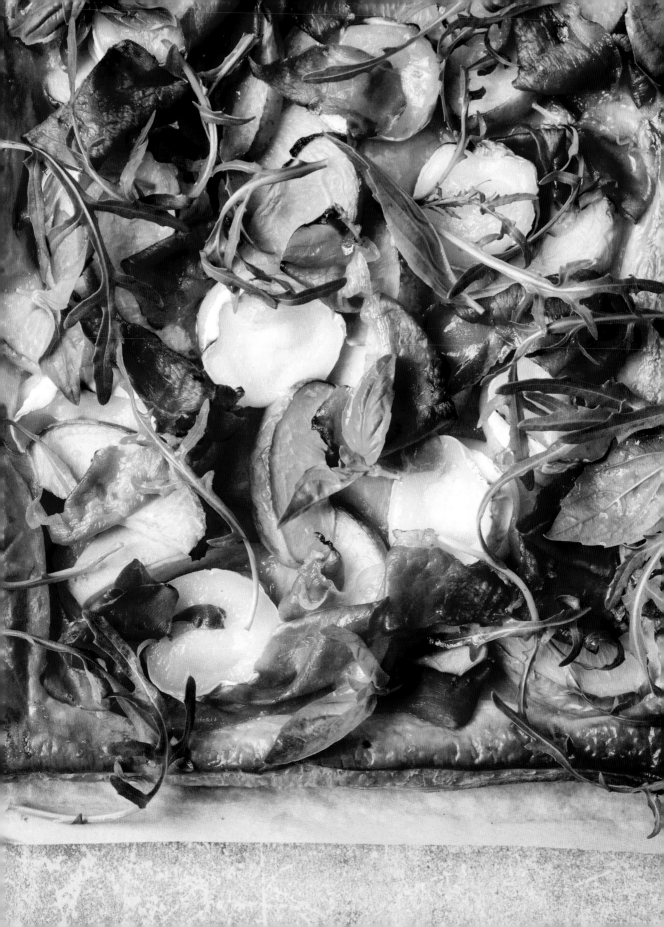

Red onion and beetroot tarte tatin

Who says a tarte tatin is just for pudding? With their rich sweet flavours, beets and red onions make good partners and they're lovely in a buttery tarte tatin – or upside down tart if you prefer. We use those packs of cooked beetroot which makes this little treat very easy to prepare.

Serves 4

1 x 320g all-butter puff pastry sheet

30g butter

2 red onions, sliced into thin wedges

1 tbsp light soft brown sugar

1 tbsp sherry vinegar

large thyme sprig, leaves only

400g cooked beetroots, cut into wedges (vac-packed are fine)

salt and black pepper

To serve
thyme leaves

a few slices of goats' cheese (optional)

Preheat the oven to 200°C/Fan 180°C/Gas 6. Take the sheet of pastry and cut it to fit an ovenproof or cast-iron frying pan with a diameter of about 20cm. The pastry should be the size of the edges, rather than the base, and larger rather than smaller. Chill the pastry until you are ready to cook the tarte tatin.

Heat the butter in the pan. When it has melted, add the red onions and cook over a medium to low heat until they have started to soften. Turn up the heat a little and add the sugar and vinegar. Stir to dissolve the sugar – a caramel-like sauce will form around the onions.

Sprinkle in the thyme, then add the wedges of beetroot. Season with plenty of salt and pepper, then stir to coat the beetroots with the buttery sauce. Make sure the beetroots are spread evenly across the pan in a single layer, then turn off the heat. Leave to cool to room temperature.

Cover the onions and beetroots with the pastry, tucking in the edges if it is a little big. Bake for 20–25 minutes until the pastry is puffed up. Remove the tart from the oven and leave to stand for 10 minutes, then invert it on to a large plate.

Sprinkle with more thyme leaves, cut into wedges, and add a slice of cheese to each slice, if using.

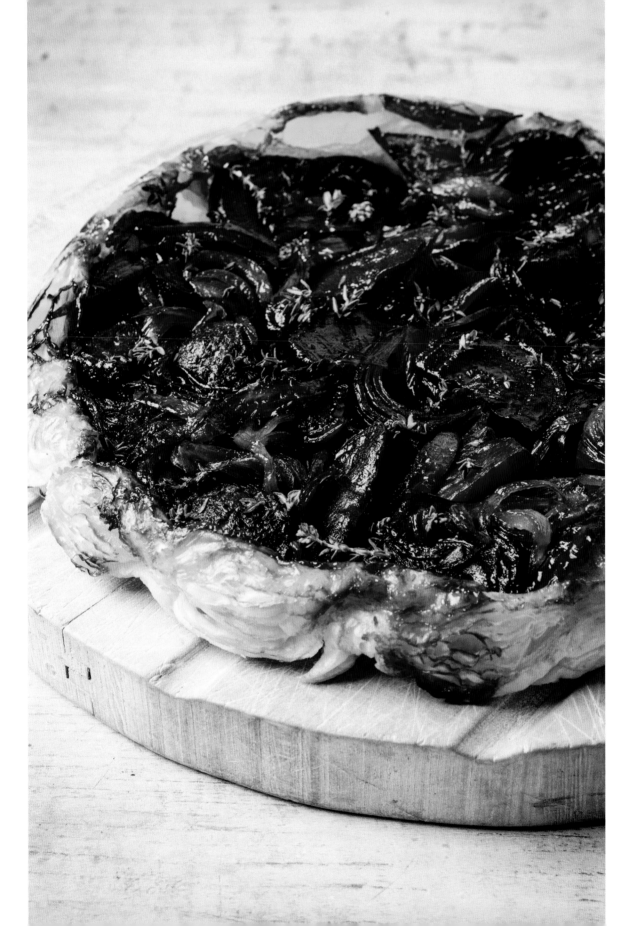

Roast vegetables with chickpeas and halloumi

Plenty of veg, carbs and protein in this trayful of Mediterranean magic. Halloumi is perfect for this sort of dish and we've discovered there are some brands available with added mint or chilli, which we rather like. See what you think.

Serves 4

2 red onions, cut into wedges

1 large red pepper, cut into thick strips

1 large green pepper, cut into thick strips

2 courgettes, diagonally sliced

2 tbsp olive oil

leaves from a rosemary sprig, finely chopped

1 tsp dried thyme

2 x 400g cans of chickpeas, drained and rinsed

juice of ½ lemon

225g block of halloumi, sliced

100g cherry tomatoes

100g rocket leaves

salt and black pepper

Preheat the oven to 200°C/Fan 180°C/Gas 6. Put all the vegetables in a large roasting tin and drizzle them with a tablespoon of the oil. Season with salt and pepper and sprinkle over the rosemary and thyme. Roast in the oven for 25 minutes.

Stir the chickpeas through the vegetables and pour over the lemon juice, then put the tin back in the oven and cook for 10 minutes. Add the halloumi and cherry tomatoes, drizzle with the remaining oil and cook for another 10 minutes. The halloumi and the chickpeas should be lightly browned, the tomatoes softened and ready to burst, and the vegetables tender and lightly charred in places.

Add the rocket to the pan and let it wilt down in the heat, then serve.

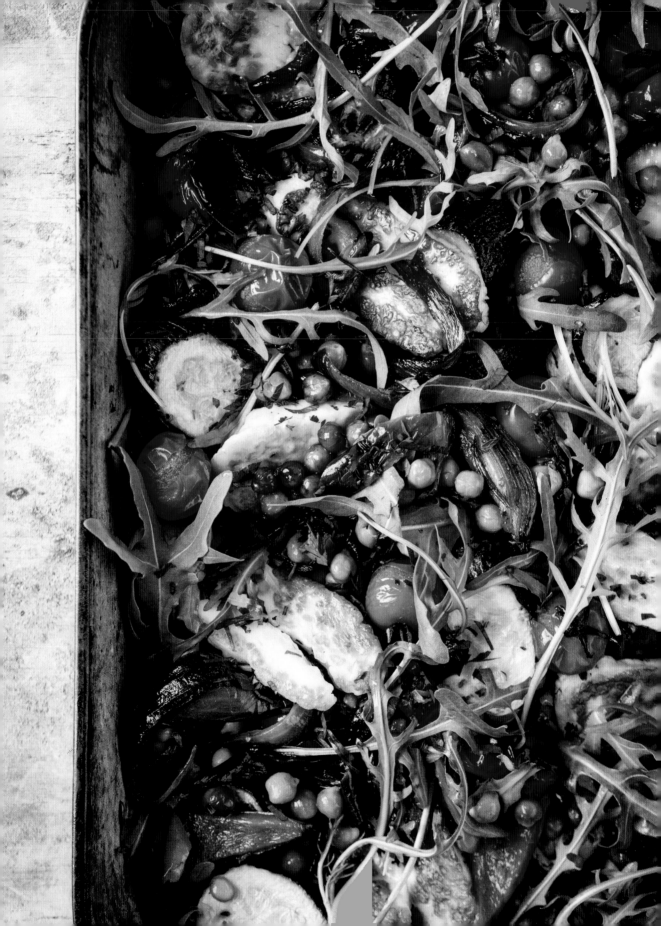

Mackerel and potato tray bake

Si has a mania for mackerel and rightly so – it's cheap, good for us and great to eat. It goes really well with potatoes and beetroot, so we've put everything together in one tasty tray bake. This is an easy dish to put together and makes a perfect mid-week supper.

Serves 4

8 mackerel fillets
1 tbsp olive oil
zest of ½ lemon
salt and black pepper

Vegetables

600g salad potatoes, halved
2 onions, sliced
2 tbsp olive oil
juice of ½ lemon
100ml white wine
1 tbsp wholegrain mustard
4 cooked beetroots, cut into
  wedges (vac-packed are
  fine)
200g cherry tomatoes, left
  whole
small bunch of dill, finely
  chopped

Check the mackerel fillets for any pin bones along the spine and remove them with tweezers. Mix the olive oil and lemon zest with plenty of seasoning and rub this over the fillets. Set them aside.

Preheat the oven to 200°C/Fan 180°C/Gas 6. Put the potatoes and onions in a large roasting tin. Drizzle over the oil, lemon juice and white wine and season generously with salt and pepper. Mix thoroughly, then roast the vegetables in the oven for half an hour. Check the potatoes – they should be almost tender but if they seem particularly firm, put them back in the oven for another 10 minutes.

Turn the oven up to 220°C/Fan 200°C/Gas 7. Stir in the mustard, then tuck in the beetroot wedges. Dot over the cherry tomatoes, then arrange the mackerel fillets on top, skin-side up. Put the tin back in the oven and cook for another 10 minutes until the mackerel is looking crisp and is piping hot. The tomatoes should feel soft, plump and ready to burst. Sprinkle with chopped dill and serve.

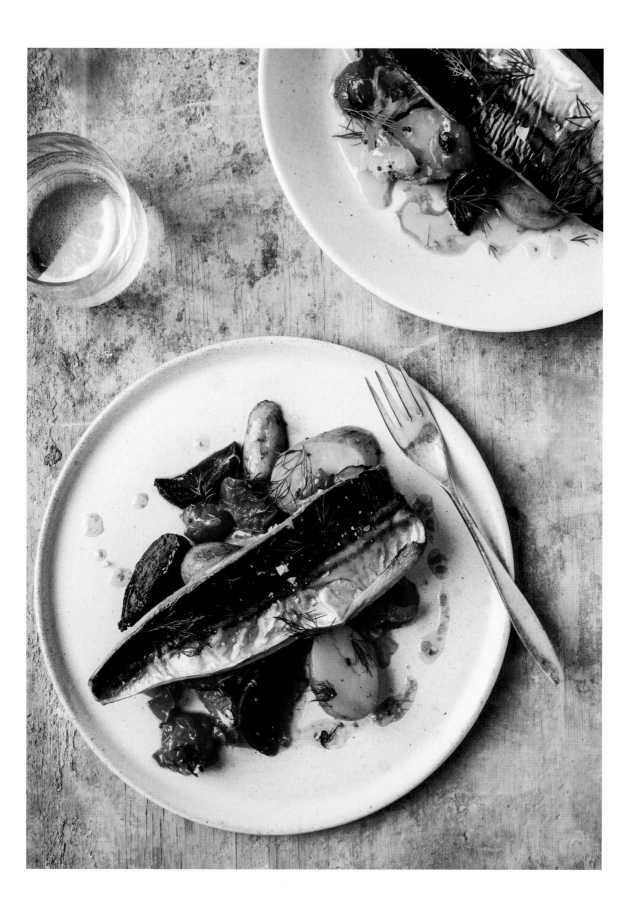

Salmon tray bake

We're told we should eat oily fish at least once a week and with recipes like this, it's no hardship. Salmon is good with a touch of sweetness, and with Asian flavours like soy sauce, so we hope you enjoy this tray bake. Kicap manis, or kepjap manis, is an Indonesian version of soy sauce, but sweeter and more syrupy. It adds a great flavour and you can buy it in most supermarkets, but if you don't have any, use honey instead.

Serves 4–6

2 red onions, cut into wedges

2 sweet potatoes, cut into large chunks

2 red peppers, cut into strips

2 tbsp sesame or olive oil

1 head of broccoli, cut into florets

400g tin of black beans, drained and rinsed

1 tbsp soy sauce

1 tbsp rice wine

2 garlic cloves, crushed

5g fresh root ginger, grated

½ tsp Chinese 5-spice powder

salt and black pepper

Salmon

600g skinned salmon fillet, cut into large chunks

1 tbsp soy sauce

1 tsp kicap manis or honey

To serve

1 tbsp sesame seeds

fresh coriander, chopped

sriracha chilli sauce, or similar

Preheat the oven to 200°C/Fan 180°C/Gas 6. Put the onions, sweet potatoes and red peppers in a roasting tin and drizzle over a tablespoon of the oil. Mix thoroughly and season with salt and pepper. Roast the veg for 20 minutes.

Toss the broccoli in the rest of the oil and add it to the roasting tin. Mix the beans with the soy sauce, rice wine, garlic, ginger and 5-spice, then add 100ml of water. Pour all this around the vegetables and cook for another 20 minutes. Turn over the broccoli once during this time if it is looking brown.

Finally, toss the salmon in the soy sauce and kicap manis or honey and place the chunks on top of the vegetables. Roast for another 8–9 minutes until the salmon is cooked – it is fine if it is slightly pink in the middle.

Serve sprinkled with sesame seeds and coriander and put a bottle of sriracha on the table for people to add if they like.

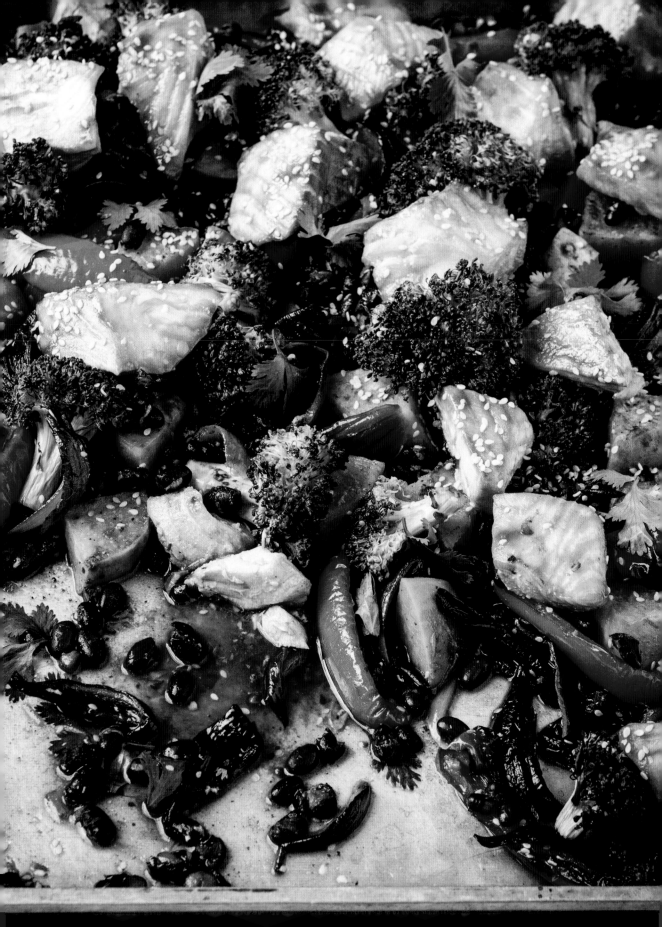

Summer chicken bake

Chicken is great in a tray bake, as the skin goes lovely and crispy and none of the tasty juices are wasted. Reminds us of summer holidays this one, with all the lovely Mediterranean veg. The spicy chickpea sauce is mega delicious and turns this tray bake into a real feast. Yes, there are quite a few ingredients but the prep is easy and then you just leave it all to cook. Enjoy!

Serves 4

8 boneless chicken thighs, skin on

zest of a lemon

2 red onions, cut into wedges

1 red pepper, cut into strips

1 green pepper, cut into strips

1 yellow pepper, cut into strips

1 tsp dried thyme

1 tsp dried oregano

2 tbsp olive oil

1 courgette, cut into rounds

salt and black pepper

Sauce

400g can of chickpeas

50ml chicken stock

juice of a lemon

3 garlic cloves, crushed

1 tsp ground cumin

1 tsp ground coriander

1 tsp ground cardamom

½ tsp ground turmeric

½ tsp cinnamon

To finish

50g black olives, pitted

100g cherry tomatoes

100g baby spinach leaves

chopped parsley

Preheat the oven to 200°C/Fan 180°C/Gas 6.

Rub the chicken with plenty of salt and the lemon zest. Spread the onions and peppers over the base of a large roasting tin and arrange the chicken thighs on top. Sprinkle with the herbs and the olive oil.

Put the tin in the oven and cook for 40 minutes. Mix the chickpeas with the stock, lemon juice, garlic and spices and season with salt and pepper. Pour this mixture around the chicken thighs and add the courgette rounds, then cook for another 15 minutes.

Add the olives and tomatoes to the tin and put it back in the oven for 5 minutes. Remove the tin and add the spinach leaves, moving the chicken thighs on top of them to help the leaves wilt down, then leave to stand for 5 minutes. Sprinkle with chopped parsley before serving.

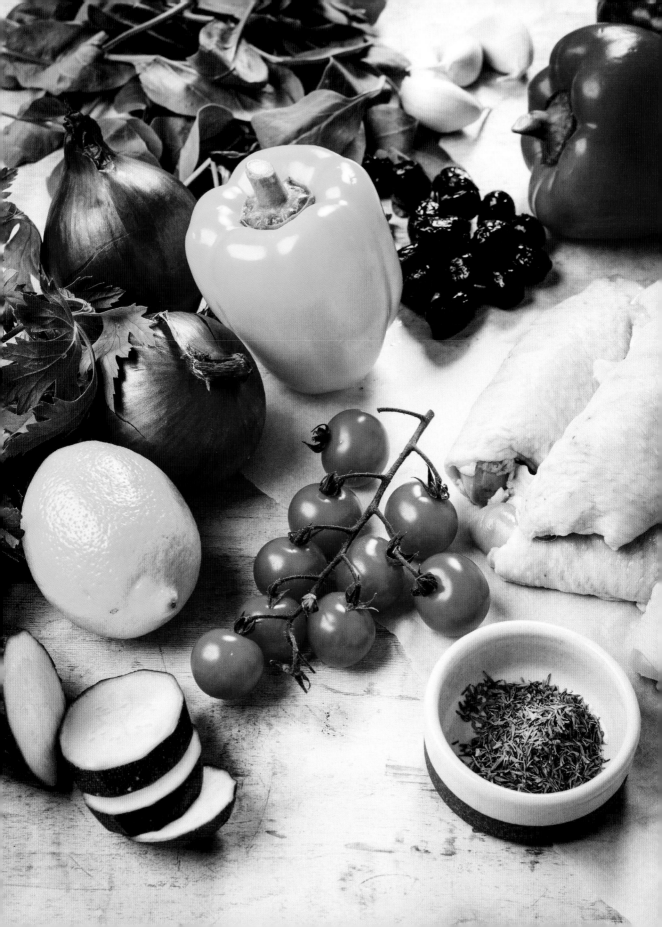

Winter chicken bake

Tray bakes are good in winter as well as summer and in this version we've used lots of good wintery vegetables such as parsnips and Brussels sprouts – almost like a Christmas dinner! The mint leaves add a nice touch of freshness at the end.

Serves 4

2–3 carrots, quartered lengthways

2–3 parsnips, quartered lengthways

3 leeks, trimmed and cut into rounds

200g Brussels sprouts, trimmed and halved

3 tbsp olive oil

8 chicken thighs, bone in, skin on

200ml white wine

1 tbsp wholegrain mustard

1 tbsp sherry vinegar

1 tsp honey

2 tsp dried thyme

300g frozen peas, defrosted

salt and black pepper

To serve
mint leaves

Preheat the oven to 200°C/Fan 180°C/Gas 6. Arrange the carrots, parsnips, leeks and Brussels sprouts in a large roasting tin and season with salt and pepper. Drizzle over half the olive oil and rub it into the vegetables, then rub the rest into the skin of the chicken thighs. Season the chicken thighs with salt and pepper and place them on top of the vegetables.

Mix the white wine with the mustard, vinegar and honey and pour it around the chicken thighs. Sprinkle the thyme over the top, then put the tin in the oven and roast for 30 minutes, stirring the vegetables once.

Remove the tin from the oven and pour in the peas around the chicken, pushing them under the vegetables as much as you can. Put the tin back in the oven for another 25–30 minutes or until the chicken is crisp and completely cooked through, and the vegetables are just tender. Serve sprinkled with fresh mint leaves.

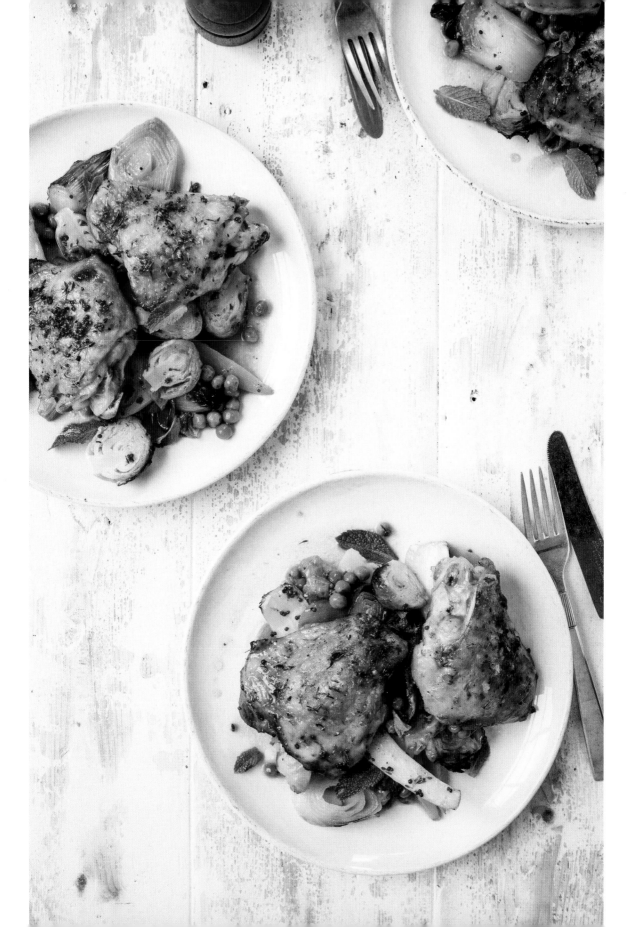

Sausage and bean supper

As kids, we both used to love those little tins of beans and sausages and here's a grown-up version in a tray bake! The bacon and the barbecue sauce give the dish a wonderful smoky savoury aroma that we know is going to get your mouth watering. We believe British sausages are some of the best in the world and this recipe is a great way of showing them off.

Serves 4

8 fat sausages

2 onions, cut into wedges

300g butternut squash, cut into thick slices

100g smoked bacon lardons

1 tsp rubbed sage

1 tbsp olive oil

2 x 400g cans of haricot beans, drained and rinsed

250ml passata

1 garlic clove, crushed

2 tbsp barbecue sauce

generous dash of Worcestershire sauce

salt and black pepper

Preheat the oven to 200°C/Fan 180°C/Gas 6. Put the sausages, onions, squash and bacon lardons into a roasting tin. Sprinkle over the sage and season with salt and pepper, then drizzle with the olive oil. Roast in the oven for 30 minutes, by which time the onions and squash should be soft and browning around the edges and the sausages will have developed a brown crust underneath.

Turn the sausages over. Mix the beans, passata, garlic, barbecue sauce and Worcestershire sauce together and season with salt and pepper. Pour this around the sausages, then stir, making sure the onions, bacon and squash are not stuck to the bottom of the tin.

Put the tin back in the oven for another 20 minutes. The sauce will have reduced around the beans a little and will be bubbling and delicious.

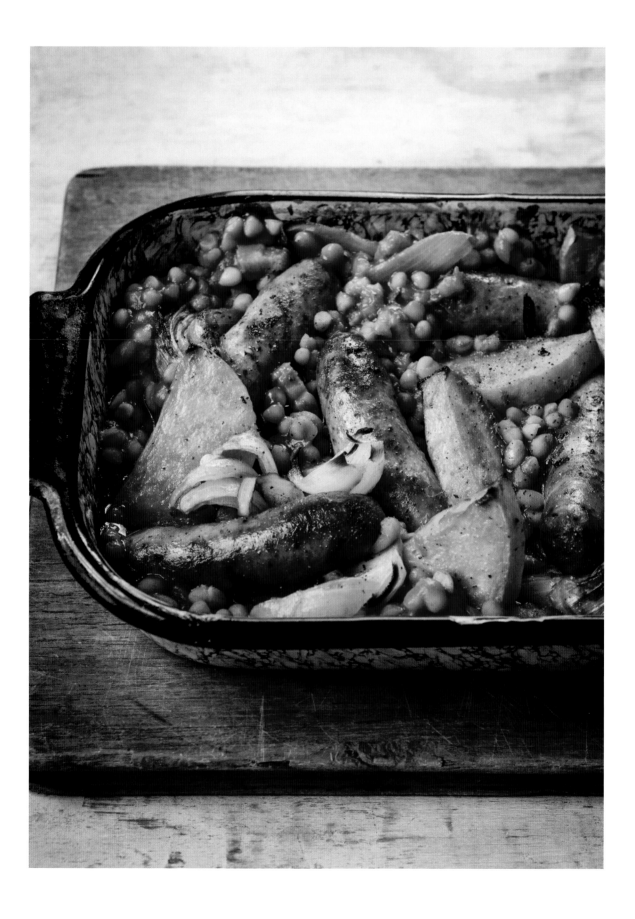

Minty lamb steaks

Lamb steaks are a really useful cut of meat, readily available and easy to prepare. They work well as a tray bake, and if you want to cut down your meat intake you could always just do two lamb steaks between four, and up the veg a little. We do think it's worth removing the skins from the broad beans to reveal their beautiful bright green colour, but if you run out of time, don't worry. Tantalisingly tasty, this one.

Serves 4

Lamb
2 tbsp olive oil
1 tbsp lemon juice
2 garlic cloves, crushed
1 tsp dried mint
4 lamb leg steaks
salt and black pepper

Vegetables
500g baby new potatoes, sliced
500g broad beans (podded weight), skinned if you have time
8 shallots, halved
2 courgettes, cut into chunks
2 tbsp olive oil
75ml white wine

To serve
chopped dill

First marinate the lamb. Mix the oil, lemon juice, garlic and mint in a bowl and add plenty of seasoning. Add the lamb steaks and rub the mixture into them. Set aside while you prepare the vegetables.

Preheat the oven to 200°C/Fan 180°C/Gas 6. Put the potatoes, broad beans, shallots and courgettes into a large roasting dish, then drizzle over the olive oil and white wine. Stir everything together, then cover the tin with foil. Roast in the oven for 30 minutes, then remove the foil and cook for another 15 minutes.

Turn the oven up to 220°C/Fan 200°C/Gas 7. Arrange the lamb steaks over the vegetables and put the tin back in the oven for 10 minutes. Remove and leave to stand for 5 minutes, then sprinkle with dill and serve.

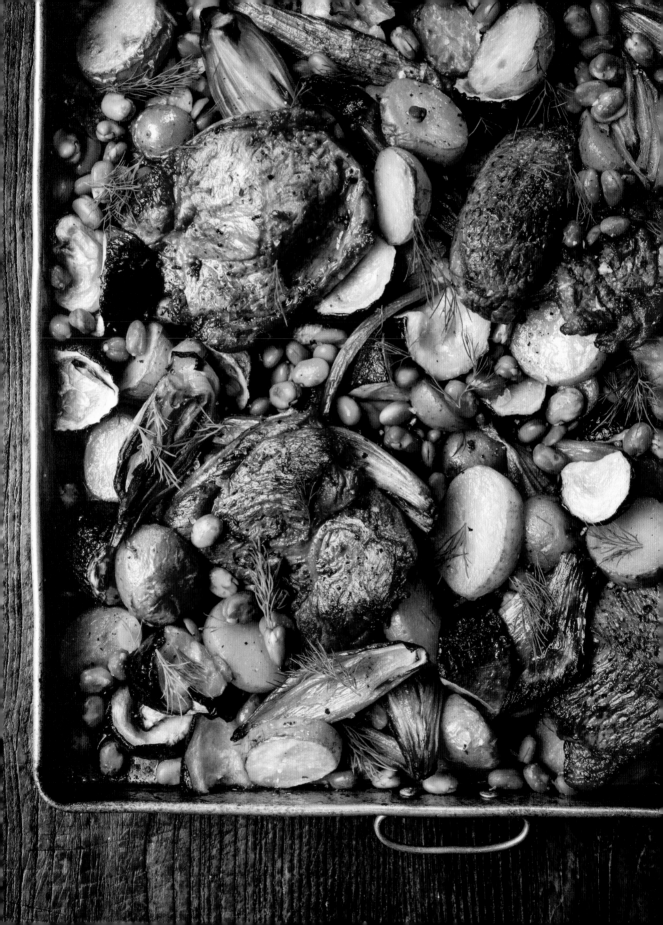

Meatball and pasta tray bake

As you all know, we're big fans of a meatball, so we had to find a way of making them into a one pot. We think this dish is heaven – meatballs, pasta, veg and sauce, all in one tin, and it tastes fab. You might wonder about the milk, but we promise you it really works. It sweetens and enriches the sauce which might otherwise be a bit acidic, as the tomatoes aren't cooked before adding. It also helps to thicken the sauce.

Serves 4

Meatballs

400g minced beef
50g breadcrumbs
50g single cream
25g Parmesan cheese, grated
2 garlic cloves, crushed
1 tsp dried oregano
salt and black pepper

Bake

1 tbsp olive oil
1 onion, finely chopped
300g short pasta, such as
  fusilli
100ml white wine
400g can of tomatoes
1 red chilli, finely chopped or
  1 tsp chilli powder
1 tsp oregano
2 garlic cloves, crushed
500ml milk
200g sprouting broccoli
1 mozzarella ball
a few basil leaves

Preheat the oven to 220°C/Fan 200°C/Gas 7. Mix all the meatball ingredients together well and season with salt and pepper. Divide into 8 balls.

Put the olive oil in a large roasting tin or a shallow cast-iron oven dish and stir in the onion. Arrange the meatballs over the base of the tin or dish and bake for 10 minutes. Meanwhile, put the pasta, wine, tomatoes, chilli or chilli powder, oregano and garlic in a bowl, season with salt and pepper and mix thoroughly.

Remove the tin from the oven and turn the oven down to 200°C/Fan 180°C/Gas 6. Pour the pasta mix around the meatballs and stir to combine with the onions. Arrange the broccoli on top, then pour in the milk. Cover the tin or dish tightly with foil, preferably 2 layers, then bake in the oven for 45 minutes.

Remove the foil and give the pasta a stir. Break up the mozzarella and arrange it over the top, add a few basil leaves, then put the dish back in the oven for another 10 minutes or until the mozzarella is melted and bubbling. Remove from the oven and leave to stand for 5 minutes before serving.

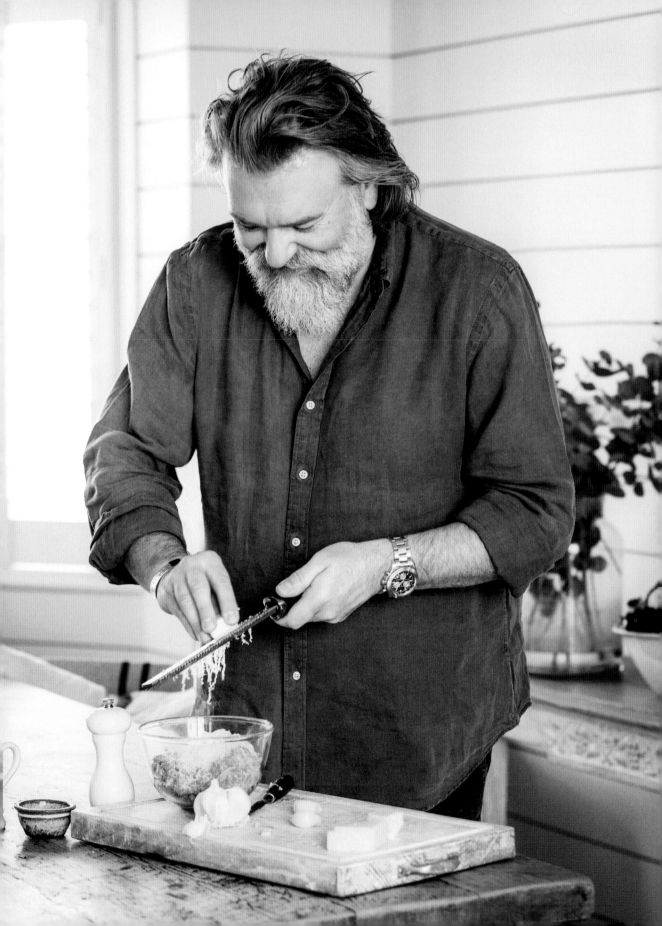

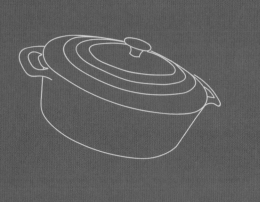
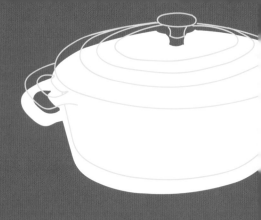
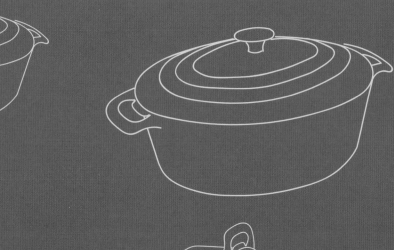

Stovetop Suppers

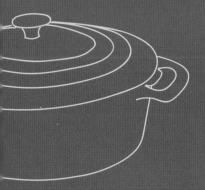
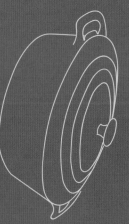
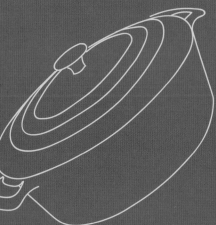

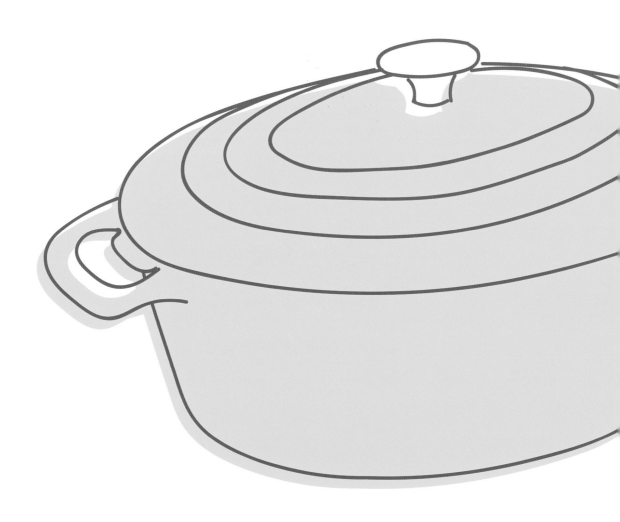

Veggie chilli with cornmeal dumplings 156

Cod, pea and potato casserole 158

Cod with chorizo and white beans 160

Fab fish and squid stew 162

Braised chicken and chicory 163

Chicken and new potato tagine 164

Duck stir-fry 166

Keema peas 168

Sausage and lentil casserole 170

Biker goulash with dumplings 172

Hearty ham hock 174

Romanian sausage bake 176

Pork and sauerkraut 178

Uzbek plov (lamb and rice to you) 180

French lamb casserole 182

Veggie chilli with cornmeal dumplings

We do like a dumpling and these sweetcorn ones are just right with our veggie chilli. There are lots of great flavours here and this is a good filling feast for hungry hordes.

Serves 4

2 tbsp olive oil

1 large onion, diced

1 green pepper, diced

1 red pepper, diced

2 celery sticks, diced

2 jalepeño chillies, finely diced

4 garlic cloves, crushed

2 bay leaves

1 tbsp ground cumin

25g red lentils, well rinsed

750ml vegetable stock

400ml coconut milk

1 head of baby spring greens, shredded

2 x 400g cans of black or pinto beans, drained and rinsed

juice of 1 lime

salt and black pepper

Cornmeal dumplings

150g self-raising flour

75g chilled butter, diced

125g fine cornmeal

125g sweetcorn, defrosted if frozen

50ml buttermilk

1 egg

To serve

100g vegetarian Cheddar cheese, grated

chopped fresh coriander

Heat the oil in a large flameproof casserole dish with a lid and add the onion, peppers, celery and chillies. Cook over a medium heat until the vegetables have started to soften, then stir in the garlic, bay leaves, cumin and red lentils. Season generously with salt and pepper, then pour in the vegetable stock.

Bring to the boil and leave for 5 minutes, then turn down the heat and continue to simmer until the red lentils have softened. Add the coconut milk, spring greens and beans and cook until the spring greens are tender and the lentils have collapsed and thickened the sauce. Taste for seasoning and add the lime juice.

To make the dumplings, put the flour into a bowl with a pinch of salt. Rub in the butter until the mixture resembles fine breadcrumbs, then mix in the cornmeal, sweetcorn, buttermilk and egg. Bring everything together into a firm dough, then divide into 12 pieces. Roll them into balls.

Arrange the dumplings over the chilli and cover. Cook over a medium heat for about 25 minutes until the dumplings are well risen and glossy. Serve the chilli with grated cheese and plenty of chopped coriander.

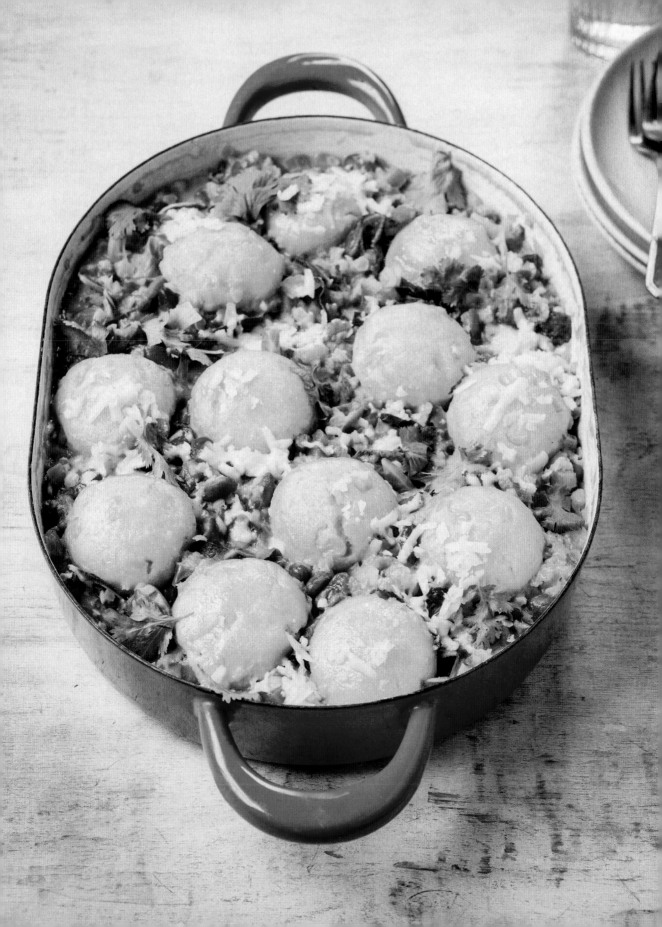

Cod, pea and potato casserole

Thick cuts of cod work really well in a casserole. We know that some people get anxious about cooking fish but this cod dish couldn't be simpler. It's easy to put together, doesn't take long to cook and it tastes epic. This is a keeper, we reckon.

Serves 4

25g butter
400g baby potatoes, halved
3 leeks, sliced
2 tarragon sprigs, left whole
100ml white wine
200ml fish or chicken stock
100ml double cream
150g peas, defrosted if frozen
4 cod fillets
salt and black pepper

Heat the butter in a large lidded sauté pan or a flameproof casserole dish, then add the potatoes and leeks. Season with salt and pepper and cook for a few minutes, turning the potatoes and leeks regularly so everything is completely coated in butter.

Add the tarragon sprigs to the pan and pour in the white wine. Turn up the heat and bring to the boil and cook for 5 minutes. Add the stock and bring it to the boil, then cover the pan and turn down the heat. Simmer until the vegetables are tender – this should take about 20 minutes.

Add the double cream and the peas, then place the cod fillets on top. Cook for a further 10–12 minutes until the cod is just cooked through. Serve piping hot.

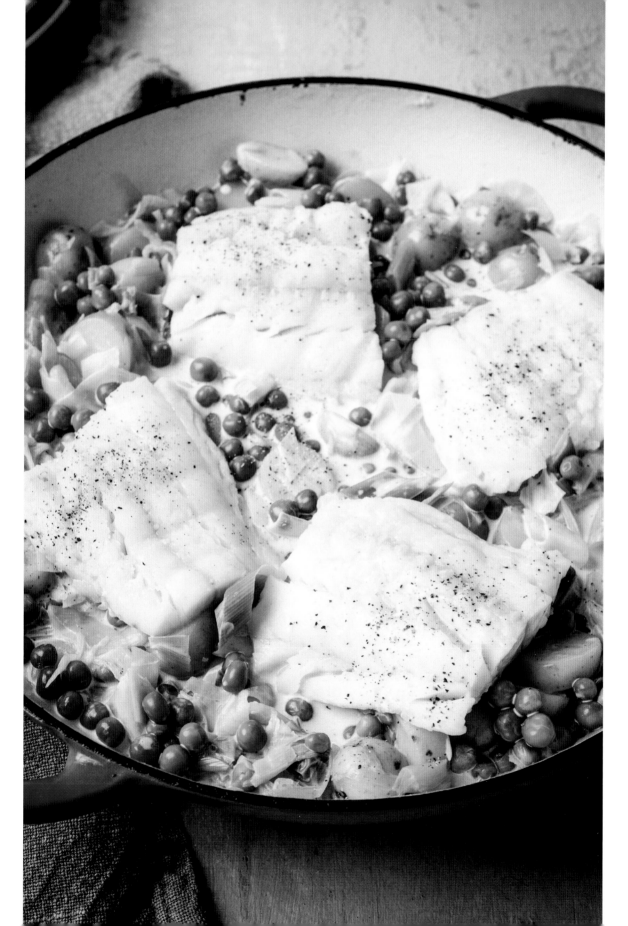

Cod with chorizo and white beans

Chorizo and red peppers give this cod dish a nice Spanish flavour. Again, this is a really easy way of cooking fish and there's plenty of delicious veg.

Serves 4

1 tbsp olive oil

150g cooking chorizo, thinly sliced

1 red onion, thinly sliced

1 red pepper, sliced

250g white cabbage, shredded

3 garlic cloves, finely chopped

1 tsp dried thyme

200ml red wine

2 tbsp tomato purée

400g can of white beans (preferably cannellini), drained and rinsed

4 cod loin steaks, skinned

salt and black pepper

To serve
chopped parsley (optional)
lemon wedges

Heat the olive oil in a large sauté pan or frying pan with a lid. Add the chorizo and brown it quickly on all sides, then remove it with a slotted spoon. If there's a lot of fat in the pan, spoon off all but about 2 tablespoons.

Add the red onion, red pepper and cabbage and cook them over a medium heat until they have started to soften, then add the garlic and thyme. Cook for a further 2–3 minutes, then turn up the heat and pour in the wine. Leave it to bubble and reduce for a couple of minutes, then stir in the tomato purée, beans and about 250ml of water. Season with salt and pepper.

Cover the pan and leave to simmer until the vegetables are just tender. Put the chorizo back in the pan. Season the cod steaks with salt and pepper and place them on top of the beans and veg. Cover the pan and leave to steam very gently for about 15 minutes or until the cod has just cooked through.

Serve sprinkled with parsley, if using, with lemon wedges on the side for squeezing over.

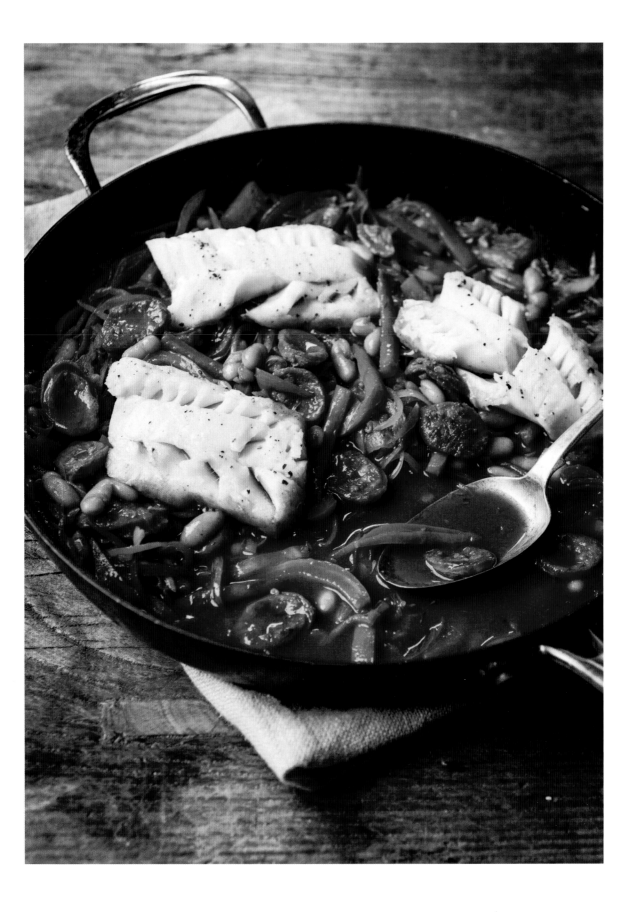

Fab fish and squid stew

Squid has become really popular in recent years and you can buy it all cleaned and ready to go. In this recipe, we combine squid with some nice white fish and plenty of veg to make a tasty stew.

Serves 4

3 tbsp olive oil

2 small fennel bulbs, each cut into 6 wedges

500g cleaned squid, cut into rings

3 garlic cloves, finely chopped

250ml white wine

large pinch of saffron, soaked in 2 tbsp warm water

bouquet garni (2 bay leaves, thyme sprig and parsley sprig)

500ml fish or chicken stock

500g baby new potatoes, halved if large

2 tomatoes, chopped

600g white fish (such as cod, hake or monkfish), cut into large chunks

salt and black pepper

To serve

finely chopped parsley or chervil

squeeze of lemon juice

Heat the olive oil in a large flameproof casserole dish. Add the fennel wedges and sear them on all sides until browned and caramelised, then remove them from the dish. Add the squid and stir fry for 2–3 minutes until lightly coloured.

Turn down the heat and add the garlic. Cook for 2 minutes, then pour in the white wine and the saffron with its soaking water. Bring to the boil for a couple of minutes, then add the bouquet garni and stock. Season with plenty of salt and pepper, then bring back to the boil, turn down the heat and cover the pan. Simmer gently for 45 minutes.

Put the fennel back in the casserole and add the potatoes. Cover again and leave for another half an hour, by which time the potatoes and fennel should be very tender.

Stir in the tomatoes, then arrange the chunks of fish on top of the vegetables. Cover and cook for a few minutes, until the fish is just done. Remove the bouquet garni and serve garnished with the chopped herbs and a squeeze of lemon juice.

Braised chicken and chicory

You can find chicory in every supermarket and it goes well with chicken in this dish. The ingredients take up a fair bit of space, so this is best cooked in a roomy pan or casserole dish. We dice the chicken to speed up the cooking time and get supper on the table quickly.

Serves 4

1 tbsp olive oil

4 skinless, boneless chicken thighs, cut into large chunks

15g butter

4 heads of chicory, trimmed and halved lengthways

2 garlic cloves, finely chopped

200g new potatoes, sliced

1 tsp rubbed sage

100ml white wine or beer

300ml chicken stock

2 tsp wholegrain mustard

200g peas, defrosted

salt and black pepper

To serve
finely chopped parsley

Heat the oil in a large sauté pan or a flameproof casserole dish. Add the chicken and cook over a high heat until the pieces are lightly browned on all sides. Remove the chicken from the pan and add the butter. When it foams, add the chicory halves, cut-side down, and cook until they are all caramelised and browned, then turn them over and cook on the other side for a few minutes. Remove the chicory from the pan and set it aside.

Add the garlic and cook for a minute or so, then add the potatoes. Stir to coat them in the buttery juices, then put the chicken back in the pan. Sprinkle in the sage and season with salt and pepper. Add the wine or beer, bring to the boil, then leave it to bubble up for a couple of minutes. Add the stock and mustard and bring back to the boil, then turn down the heat and leave to simmer, uncovered, for 10 minutes until the potatoes are almost cooked.

Put the chicory back in the pan and sprinkle in the peas. Continue to cook until the potatoes and chicory are tender to the point of a knife and the sauce has reduced to a syrupy consistency. Serve sprinkled with parsley.

Chicken and new potato tagine

We've added potatoes to our chicken tagine to make it into a good complete meal and they soak up the chicken juices beautifully. If you prefer, though, you could leave the potatoes out and serve the tagine with couscous instead. The spicing, olives and fruit give this dish a fantastic fragrant flavour.

Serves 4

2 tbsp olive oil

2 fennel bulbs, cut into wedges

300g baby new potatoes

6 skinless, boneless chicken thighs

3 garlic cloves, crushed

1 tsp ground cardamom

½ tsp ground cinnamon

½ tsp ground coriander

½ tsp ground turmeric

½ tsp cayenne

pinch of saffron, soaked in 2 tbsp warm water

500ml chicken stock

12 green olives

juice of ½ lemon

1 orange, peeled and cut into segments (see p.52)

mint leaves, to garnish

salt and black pepper

Heat the oil in a large pan. Add the fennel and potatoes and sear them on all sides until they look caramelised around the edges. Remove them from the pan.

Add the chicken thighs to the pan and sear them on all sides. Sprinkle in the garlic and spices and stir to combine, then pour in the saffron with its soaking water and the chicken stock. Put the vegetables back in the pan and add the green olives, then season with salt and pepper.

Bring to the boil, then turn down the heat and partially cover the pan. Simmer for about half an hour until the vegetables are tender. Remove from the heat and add the lemon juice and orange segments. Garnish with mint leaves, then serve.

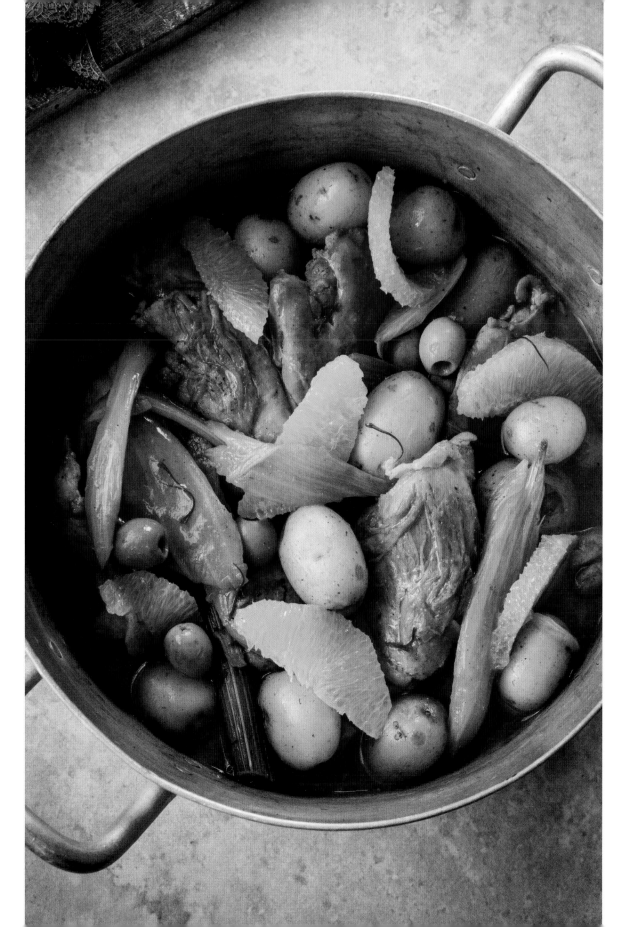

Duck stir-fry

Ooh, we love a duck! Stir-fries are the ultimate one pot for us and this recipe is super-quick to make and awesome to eat. It will disappear faster than you can say quack, quack. We use precooked noodles that you can add straight from the packet or you can cook your own if you prefer.

Serves 2–3

2 tbsp vegetable oil

4 tbsp light soy sauce

1 tbsp rice wine vinegar

1 tbsp honey

1 tsp Chinese 5-spice powder

2 skinless duck breasts, thinly sliced

1 red onion, finely sliced

1 red pepper, finely sliced

2 heads of baby spring greens, shredded

20g fresh root ginger, finely chopped

3 garlic cloves, finely chopped

300g precooked noodles

salt and black pepper

To serve

1 tsp sesame oil

2 spring onions, shredded

roughly chopped fresh coriander

Heat half the oil in a large wok. Mix together the soy sauce, rice wine vinegar, honey and 5-spice and set aside.

Season the duck with a generous amount of salt and pepper. When the air above the oil is shimmering, add the slices of duck and stir-fry for 2–3 minutes until they're well browned and just cooked through. Remove them from the wok.

Add the remaining oil to the wok. Again, when the air is shimmering, add the onion, pepper, spring greens, ginger and garlic. Stir-fry for 3–4 minutes. Then pour the soy sauce mixture into the wok with a splash of water. Cook, continuing to stir regularly, until the greens are cooked through, then put the duck back in the wok along with the noodles.

Toss everything together, then serve drizzled with sesame oil and garnished with spring onions and coriander.

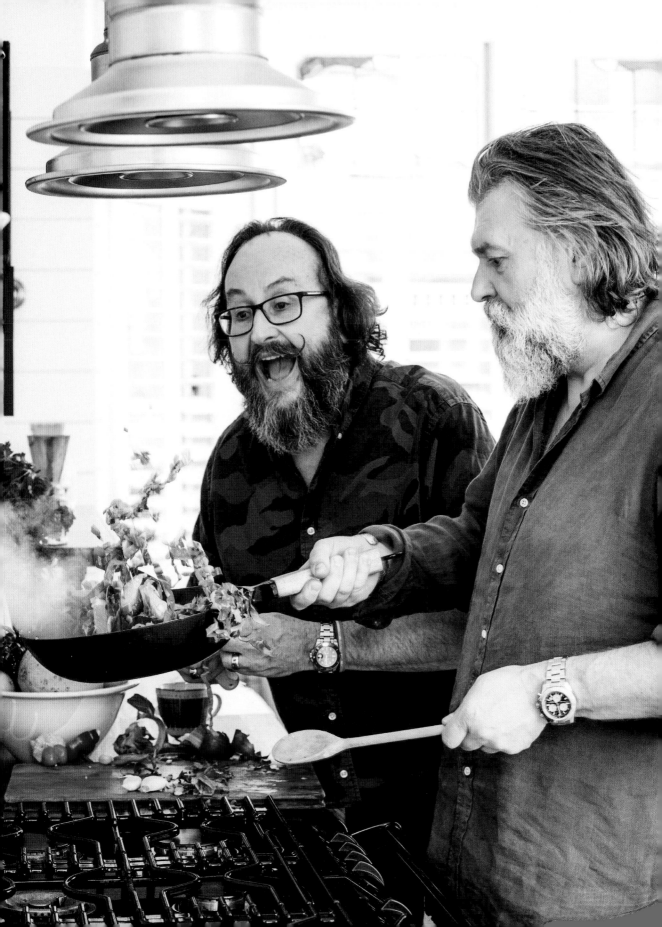

Keema peas

We northerners have a penchant for mince and peas but so do the people in northern India. This is a classic one pot and a regular in both our households. It's easy to put together and then you can just leave it to bubble away for half an hour and supper is ready. Cooking the peas for a long time like this gives them a lovely sweet softness – almost like tinned peas which we love – but if you want to keep them bright and green, just add them 5 minutes before the end of the cooking time.

Serves 4

1 tbsp vegetable oil
1 onion, finely chopped
500g lean lamb mince
15g fresh root ginger, grated
3 garlic cloves, finely chopped
small bunch of coriander
2 tbsp mild curry powder
   (shop-bought or see p.266)
1 tsp nigella seeds
2 bay leaves
200g canned tomatoes
100ml coconut milk
300g peas, defrosted
salt and black pepper

To serve
green chillies, sliced
lemon or lime wedges
flatbreads (naan or roti)

Heat the oil in a large saucepan. Add the onion and cook until soft and translucent, then turn up the heat and add the lamb. Sear until the lamb is well browned, then stir in the ginger and garlic. Separate the coriander leaves from the stems, reserve the leaves and finely chop the stems. Add the stems to the pan with the curry powder, nigella seeds and bay leaves and stir to combine.

Add the canned tomatoes, coconut milk, peas and about 100ml of water, then season with plenty of salt and pepper. Bring to the boil, then turn down the heat to a simmer and cook for about 30 minutes until the sauce has reduced and is lovely and creamy.

Garnish with the coriander leaves and green chillies and serve with some lemon or lime wedges and flatbread.

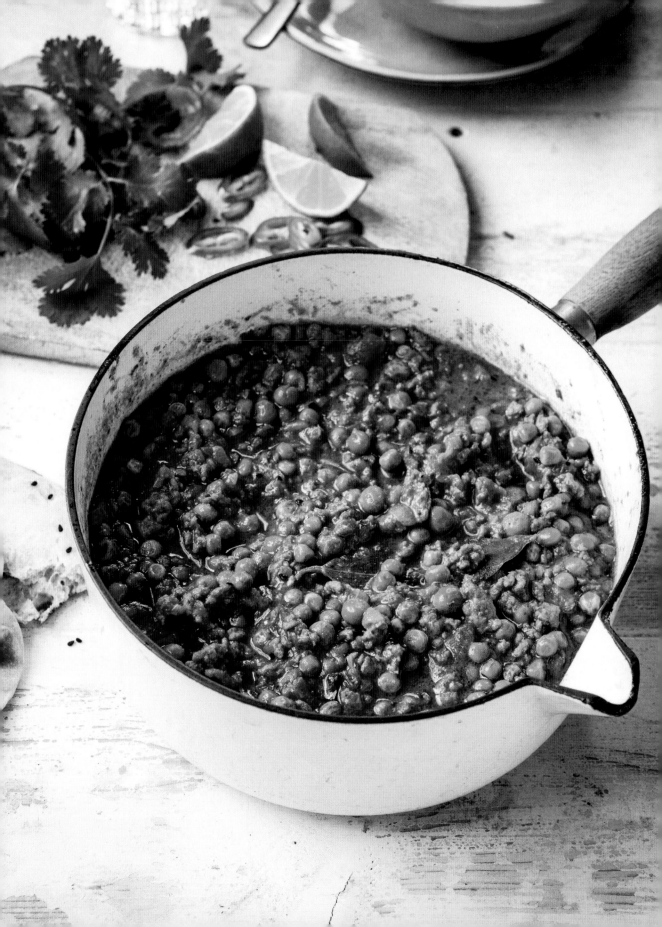

Sausage and lentil casserole

Lentils are good for you but they are also great for absorbing flavour – and in this casserole there's plenty of that. Sausages and lentils love each other and make a perfect one pot. Serve this up for tea and you'll see big smiles on everyone's face.

Makes 4

1 tbsp olive oil

8 sausages

1 onion, finely chopped

2 celery sticks, diced

1 carrot, diced

3 garlic cloves, chopped

1 thyme sprig

2 bay leaves

300g puy lentils

250ml red wine

750ml vegetable or chicken stock

1 tbsp Dijon mustard

150g green beans, trimmed and halved

salt and black pepper

To serve
chopped parsley

Heat the oil in a large flameproof casserole dish and fry the sausages over a high heat until browned on all sides. Turn down the heat and continue to cook the sausages for about 10 minutes until just cooked through. Remove them from the dish and set them aside.

Add the onion, celery and carrot to the casserole dish and cook for several minutes until the onion has started to soften. Add the garlic, thyme and bay leaves, then the lentils. Stir to coat them with the oil, then pour in the wine.

Turn up the heat and let the wine bubble up and reduce by half, then add the stock and mustard. Season with plenty of salt and pepper. Bring everything to the boil, then reduce the heat to a simmer, partially cover the dish and cook until the lentils are tender. This can take anything from half an hour to 45 minutes. Stir regularly to prevent the mixture catching on the bottom of the dish. After 20 minutes add the green beans, leaving them on the surface of the lentils so they part simmer, part steam.

When the lentils and green beans are tender, stir to mix the beans into the sauce. Put the sausages back in the dish – leave them whole or slice into chunks if you prefer. Cook for another 10 minutes until piping hot, adding a splash more liquid if necessary. Taste for seasoning and garnish with plenty of parsley.

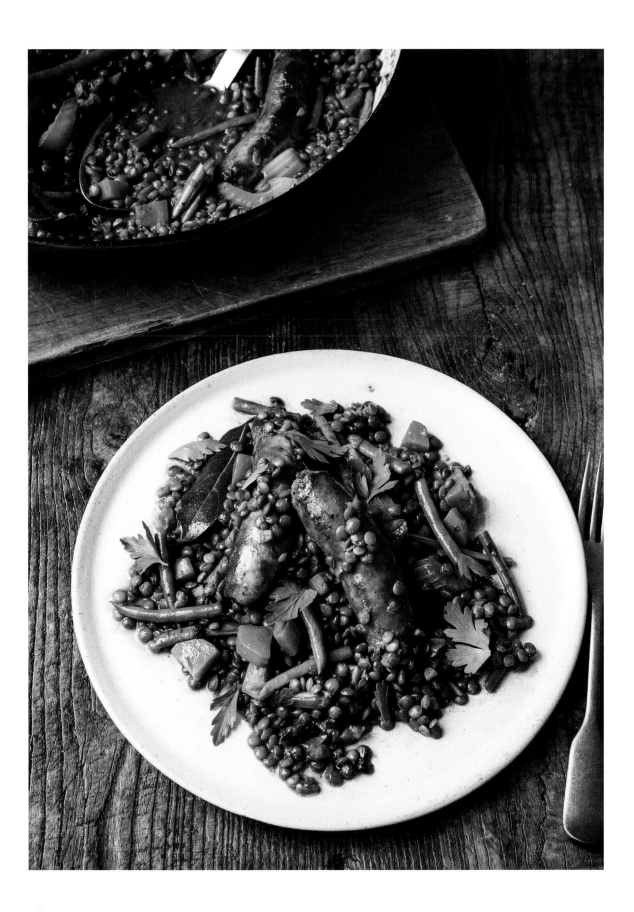

Biker goulash with dumplings

We're goofy about goulash and we've cooked many versions of it over the years. This is our latest and we hope you love it as much as we do – anything with dumplings is a winner for us. It does take a while to cook, but once it's all in the pan you can leave it to simmer and go away to practice your Hungarian dancing. And when it's ready, we promise you won't go hungry – ha, ha!

Serves 6

———

2 tbsp oil or dripping
2 red peppers, cut into slices
1 green pepper, cut into slices
750g braising steak (such as chuck), diced
2 onions, thickly sliced
1 tbsp sweet paprika
1 tsp hot paprika
2 tbsp tomato purée
3 garlic cloves, crushed
600ml beef stock
1 bay leaf
salt and black pepper

Dumplings
200g self-raising flour
100g suet

To serve
soured cream

Heat a tablespoon of the oil or dripping in a large flameproof casserole dish or a saucepan. Add the peppers and cook them over a high heat until the skins are starting to brown. Remove them from the pan, add the meat and sear it over a high heat until browned on all sides. Remove the meat and set it aside.

Warm the rest of the oil or dripping in the pan, add the onions and cook them over a medium heat until they're starting to soften and take on some colour, then put the beef back in the pan. Sprinkle over the paprikas, tomato purée and garlic, stir to combine and pour in the stock. Bring to the boil, turn the heat down to a simmer and add the bay leaf and plenty of seasoning. Leave to simmer for an hour.

Put the peppers back in the pan and leave to simmer for another half an hour, by which time the beef and peppers should be tender.

Meanwhile, make the dumplings. Put the flour and suet into a bowl with plenty of seasoning and add just enough cold water to form a slightly sticky dough.

When you are happy that the beef is tender, drop balls of the dumpling mixture on to the surface of the casserole. Cover with a lid and leave to cook for 20 minutes. The dumplings will puff up and look very glossy when they are done.

Serve the goulash and dumplings with spoonfuls of soured cream.

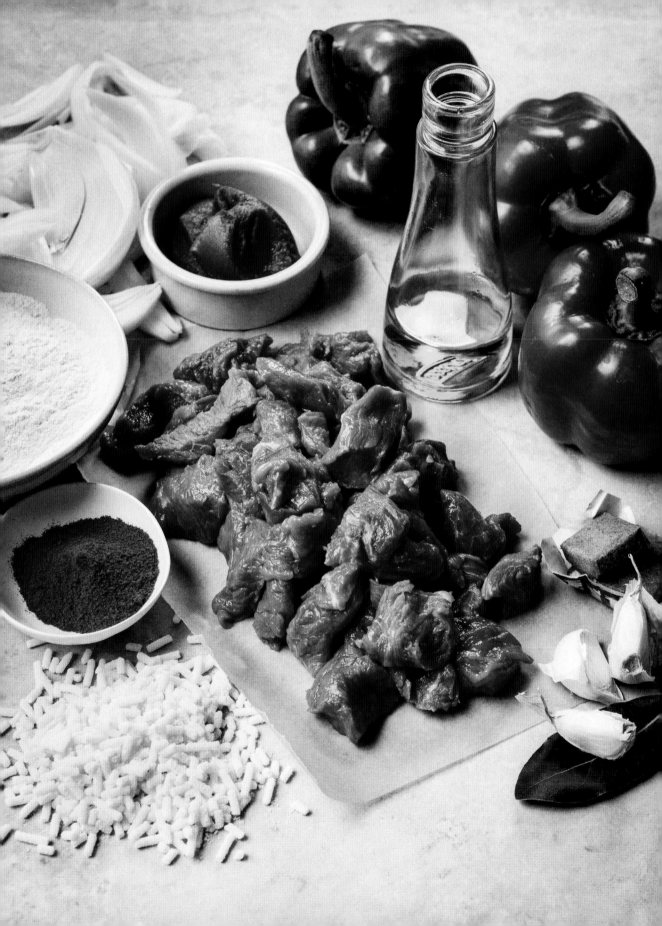

Hearty ham hock

Who doesn't love a ham hock? It's cheap and has bags of flavour that the veg absorb. This is another great one pot that takes a while to cook, but there's very little prep to do and you can leave it all simmering happily while you do other things. A good, rustic dish.

Serves 4–6

1 small ham hock or pork knuckle

1 onion, studded with 3 cloves

2 bay leaves

1 tsp allspice berries, crushed

2 onions, cut into wedges

3 carrots, cut into chunks

3 celery sticks, cut into chunks

½ celeriac, cut into chunks

2 large floury potatoes, peeled and cut into chunks

3 leeks, cut into thick rounds

½ savoy cabbage, cut into wedges

1 head of garlic

To serve
finely chopped parsley

mustard

Put the ham hock in a large pan, cover it with water and bring to the boil. Boil for 5 minutes, skimming off any foam from the surface. Take the pan off the heat, pour the water away, then rinse the ham hock and the pan.

Cover the hock with fresh water and add the onion studded with cloves, the bay leaves and allspice berries. Bring to the boil, then turn down the heat and simmer, uncovered, for about an hour and a half until the ham hock is tender. Remove the hock and the onion from the pan and leave them to cool.

Check the amount of liquid in the pan – you need about a litre. Ladle off any extra and keep it to use as stock. Add the onion wedges and other vegetables, then peel off the outer papery layers of the head of garlic and add that too. Bring to the boil, then turn the heat down and simmer until the vegetables are very tender and the potatoes have started to break up and thicken the broth. Take the garlic out and squeeze the flesh from cloves into the broth.

Remove the rind and bone from the ham hock and break the meat up into large chunks. Add the meat to the casserole and heat through. Garnish with parsley and serve with plenty of mustard.

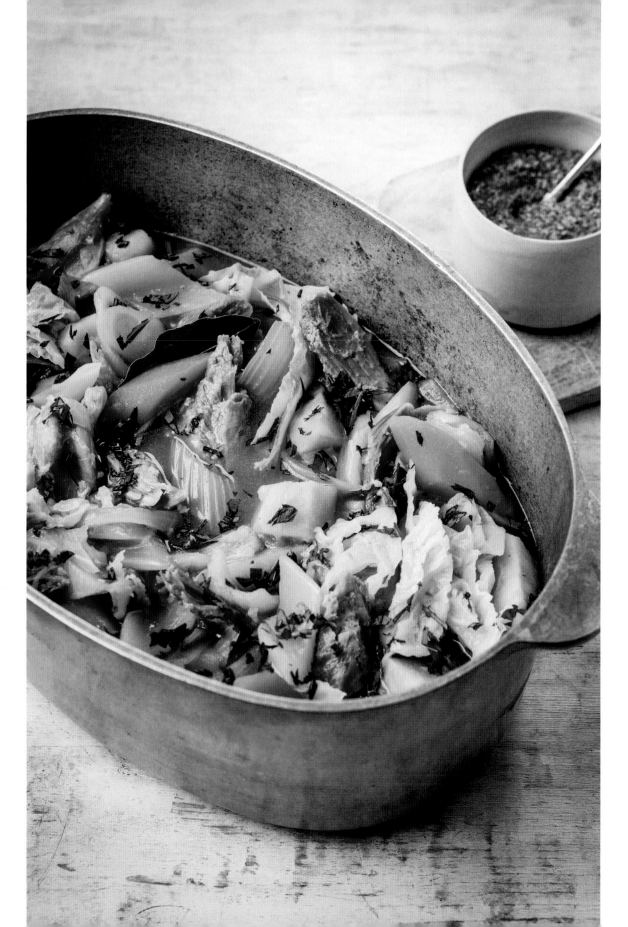

Romanian sausage bake

Dave: this is something that Lil, my wife, often cooks for me when I get back from filming. Served up with a glass of red wine, it's my guilty pleasure. We've come up with a one pot version using quick-cook polenta that thickens almost immediately. If you use regular medium-grain polenta it may take up to 20 minutes.

Serves 4

1 tbsp olive oil

150g smoked bacon, diced

200g smoked sausage (such as kielbasa), cut into rounds

2 onions, sliced into thin wedges

500ml milk

500ml chicken stock or water

200g polenta

150g Cheddar cheese, grated

salt

Preheat the oven to 200°C/Fan 180°C/Gas 6.

Heat the olive oil in a large flameproof casserole dish. Add the bacon, sausage and onions and fry them over a medium heat until everything is well browned. Remove them with a slotted spoon and set aside.

Put the milk and the stock or water in the same pan and bring to the boil, while stirring to scrape up any brown bits on the base of the pan. The liquid will have an orange tint to it.

Sprinkle in the polenta and add salt. Stir constantly until the polenta has thickened, then stir in half the cheese. Put the onions and meat back in the pan and stir them in, then sprinkle over the rest of the cheese.

Put the casserole dish in the oven and bake for about 20 minutes until the cheese is bubbling and brown in patches. Serve piping hot.

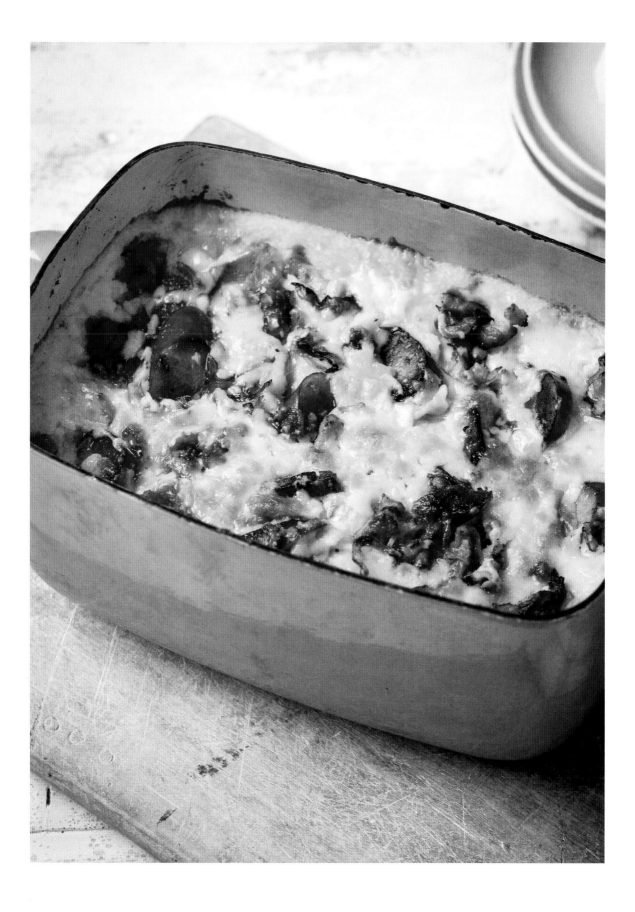

Pork and sauerkraut

We've based this on the classic Polish favourite of meat and sauerkraut known as bigos, but we've added extra greens in the form of shredded cabbage, and some potatoes to make it a one pot. It's a real rib-sticker this one – great on a cold night.

Serves 4

1 tbsp oil or lard

100g smoked bacon lardons

2 onions, finely sliced

300g pork leg, finely diced

1 tsp juniper berries

2 garlic cloves, crushed

300g drained sauerkraut

500g floury potatoes, halved and thickly sliced

400g chicken or vegetable stock or water

1 small green pointed cabbage, shredded

200g smoked sausage (such as kielbasa), cut into rounds (optional)

salt and black pepper

To serve
mustard

Heat the oil or lard in a large flameproof casserole dish or a saucepan and add the bacon and onions. Cook over a medium to high heat until the onions are lightly caramelised and the bacon has crisped up. Stir in the pork and continue to cook until the meat has browned on all sides.

Add the juniper berries, garlic, sauerkraut and potatoes to the pan and season with plenty of salt and pepper. Add the stock or water, then bring to the boil. Cover the pan, turn the heat down to a simmer and cook for an hour, until the pork is tender.

Add the cabbage and the sausage, if using, and continue to cook until the cabbage is tender – about another half an hour. Serve with plenty of mustard on the side.

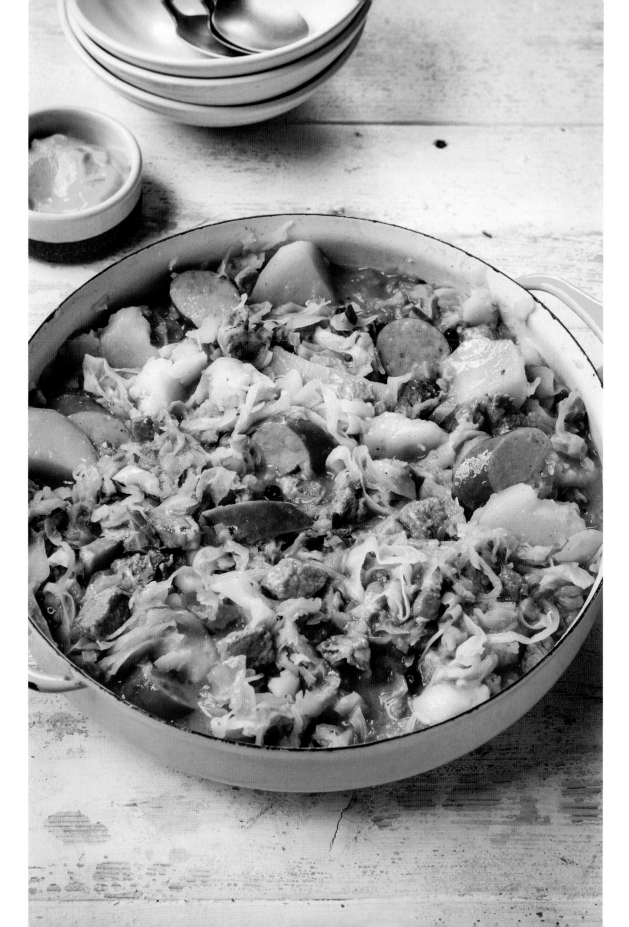

Uzbek plov (lamb and rice to you)

This dish from Uzbekistan makes an amazing one pot supper and is traditionally prepared in a special pot called a kazan over an open fire. A plov generally contains rice, meat, onions and grated or shredded carrots but every family has their own variation – we hope we haven't taken too many liberties with ours. It can be cooked in huge quantities, so is an ideal dish for a big celebration. Lamb neck fillet is a good economical cut – it's lean and tasty.

Serves 4–6

1 tbsp vegetable oil

600g lamb neck fillet, diced

2 large onions, sliced

2 carrots, shredded or coarsely grated

1 tsp cumin seeds

1 tsp coriander seeds

up to a litre of chicken or vegetable stock or water

400g basmati rice

1 head of garlic, left whole

salt and black pepper

To serve (optional)
large gherkins
pickled green chillies

Heat the oil in a large flameproof casserole dish, then add the lamb and sear it on all sides. Add the onions and carrots and continue to cook over a medium, heat, stirring regularly, until the onions have softened. The lamb does start giving out some liquid during this time.

Add the cumin and coriander seeds and season generously with salt and pepper. Pour in some of the stock or water to cover and bring to the boil, then turn the heat down and leave to simmer for about an hour until the meat is tender.

While the lamb is cooking, rinse the rice until the water runs clear, then leave it to soak in warm water for 30 minutes.

Using a slotted spoon, remove the lamb and vegetables from the casserole dish. Pour the remaining liquid into a jug and make it up to 800ml with stock or water. Put the meat and vegetables back into the dish.

Drain the rice thoroughly and add it to the dish. Stir to coat in the juices, then pour in the 800ml of stock.

Peel away the outer couple of layers of the head of garlic and trim the top with a sharp knife – just enough to take off the topmost tips of the cloves. Put the garlic head in the centre of the rice. Bring to the boil, then turn down the heat and put a lid on the casserole dish. Simmer for 15 minutes until the rice is cooked and has absorbed all the liquid, then remove the dish from the heat. Take off the lid, cover the dish with a folded tea towel and replace the lid. Leave to steam off the heat for 10 minutes.

Fluff up the rice a little and serve the plov straight from the dish, with a few gherkins and chillies if you like. Everyone can squeeze the flesh from the soft garlic cloves on to their serving.

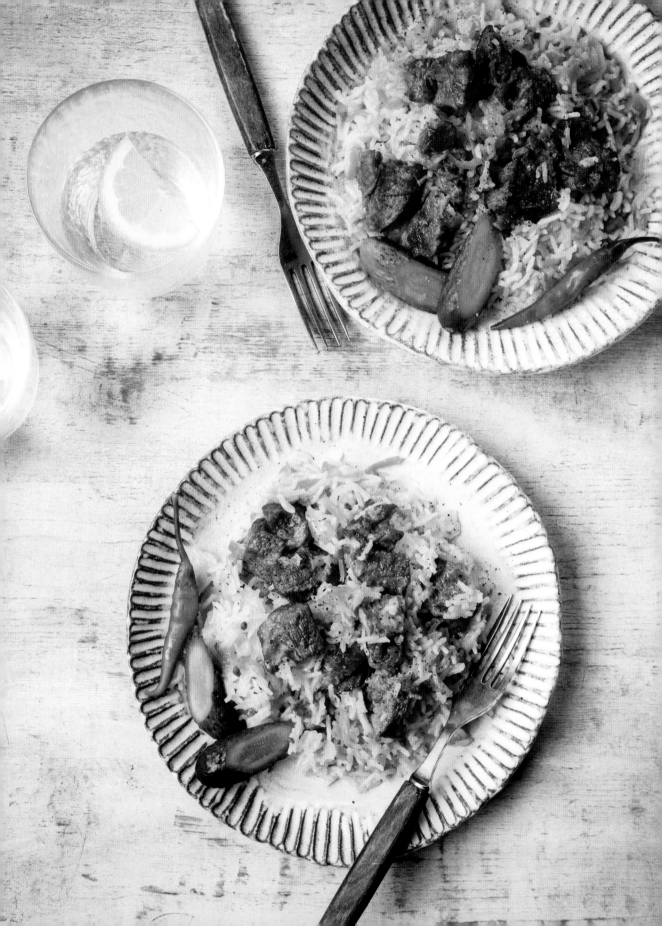

French lamb casserole

The French term for this classic lamb and vegetable stew is navarin – the name may come from the French word for turnips, 'navet', which are always part of this dish. You'll notice we include some anchovies in the ingredients but don't worry, the stew won't taste fishy. The anchovies just bring a wonderfully rich savoury flavour to the lamb and put a little joie de vivre into your supper.

Serves 4–6

2 tbsp olive oil

2 onions, cut into wedges

2 carrots, cut into fine slices

4 turnips, cut into wedges

2 leeks, cut into rounds on the diagonal

1 large courgette, cut into rounds on the diagonal

600g lamb neck fillet, cubed

4 garlic cloves, crushed

50g can of anchovies, drained and chopped

a few rosemary sprigs

1 thyme sprig

2 bay leaves

300ml white wine

200ml chicken stock

2 x 400g cans of flageolet beans, drained and rinsed

salt and black pepper

To serve
finely chopped parsley

Heat the oil in a large flameproof casserole dish. When it's really hot, add all the vegetables and cook them over a high heat until lightly browned. You can do this in a couple of batches if you like.

Remove the vegetables from the pan and add the pieces of lamb. Sear them on all sides, then stir in the garlic and anchovies. Add the herbs and season with salt and pepper, then pour in the wine. Bring to the boil and leave to bubble for 5 minutes, then add the stock. Partially cover the dish with a lid and turn down the heat. Leave to simmer for 45 minutes.

Put the vegetables back in the casserole dish and leave to cook, partially covered, for another half an hour, by which time everything should be perfectly tender. If not, cook for a few more minutes. Add the beans and cook for another 10 minutes. Check for seasoning and serve garnished with plenty of chopped parsley.

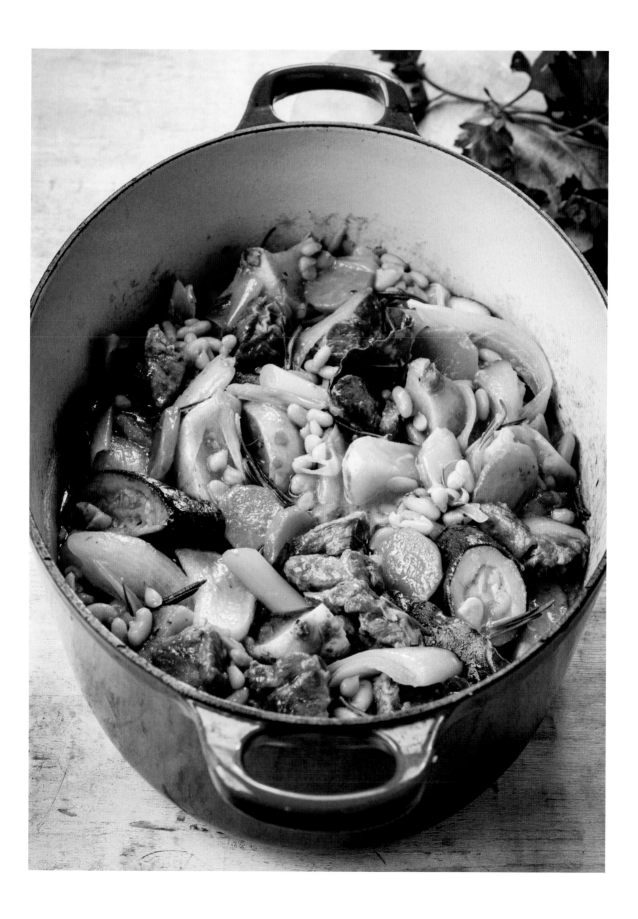

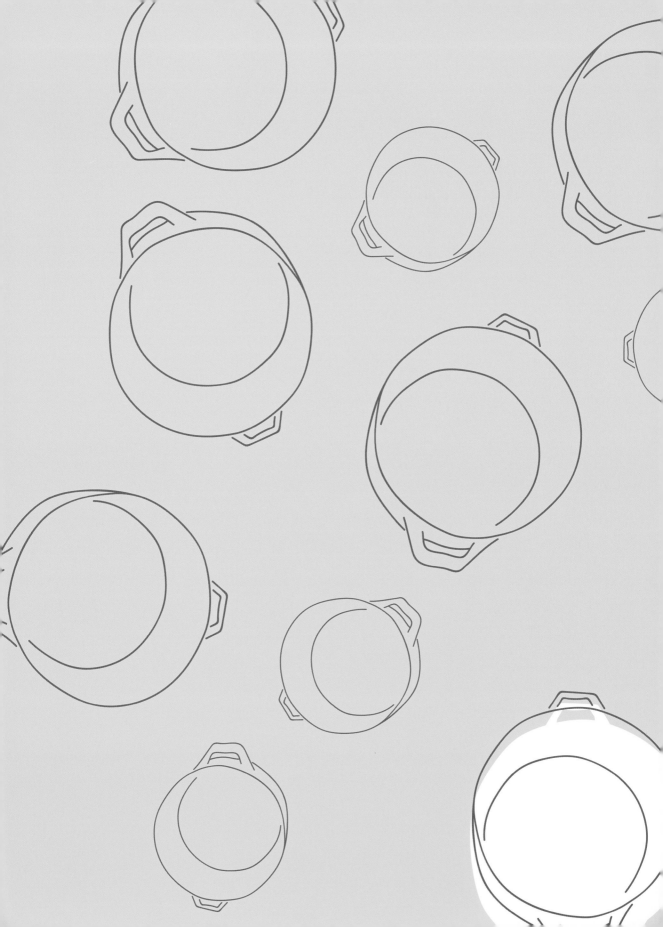

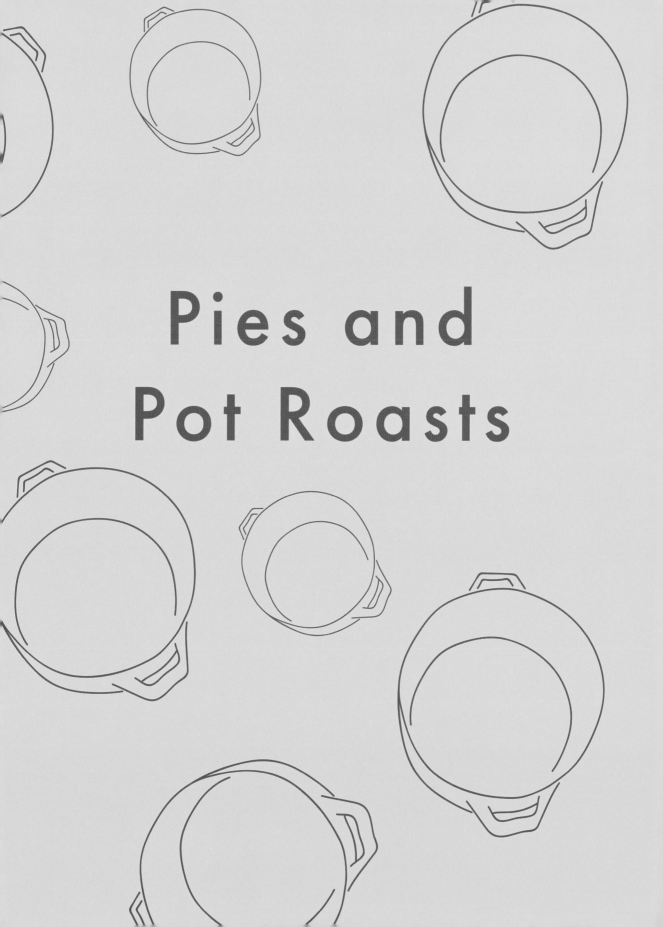

Pies and Pot Roasts

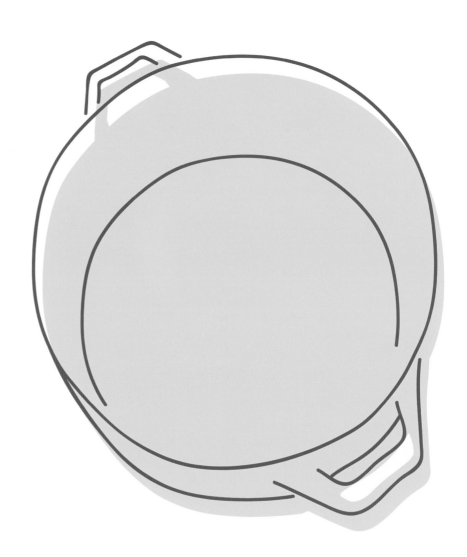

Vegetable crumble

A good old crumble topping goes just as well with a savoury filling as sweet, and this is a big favourite of ours. You can vary the veg of course, but we think this is a great combo and certainly a tasty way of having your five a day. The topping is so delicious we have to resist picking it all off before getting to the veg.

Serves 4

1 tbsp olive oil

15g butter

1 onion, diced

2 celery sticks, diced

250g mushrooms, halved if large

300g butternut squash, diced

50ml white wine

100ml vegetable stock

½ head of broccoli, cut into small florets

1 small cauliflower, cut into small florets

100ml single cream

100g vegetarian Cheddar cheese, grated

salt and black pepper

Topping

150g plain flour

75g butter, plus extra to dot on the top

small bunch of parsley, finely chopped

50g Cheddar cheese, grated

Preheat the oven to 180°C/Fan 160°C/Gas 4. Heat the olive oil and butter in a large flameproof casserole dish and add the onion and celery. Cook until the onion is soft, then turn up the heat and add the mushrooms and squash. Cook until the mushrooms are lightly browned, then pour in the white wine and allow it to bubble up. Add the stock and season with salt and pepper.

Put the broccoli and cauliflower on top of the other vegetables so they sit above the liquid, then bring to the boil. Turn down the heat, cover the dish with a lid and simmer until the vegetables are just tender. Stir in the cream and cheese.

For the crumble topping, put the flour in a bowl with salt and pepper, then rub in the butter. Stir in the parsley and cheese. Sprinkle the mixture over the vegetables then dot with a little butter.

Bake in the oven for 25–30 minutes until the crumble topping is golden brown and the vegetable sauce is bubbling up around the sides. Leave to settle for 5 minutes before serving.

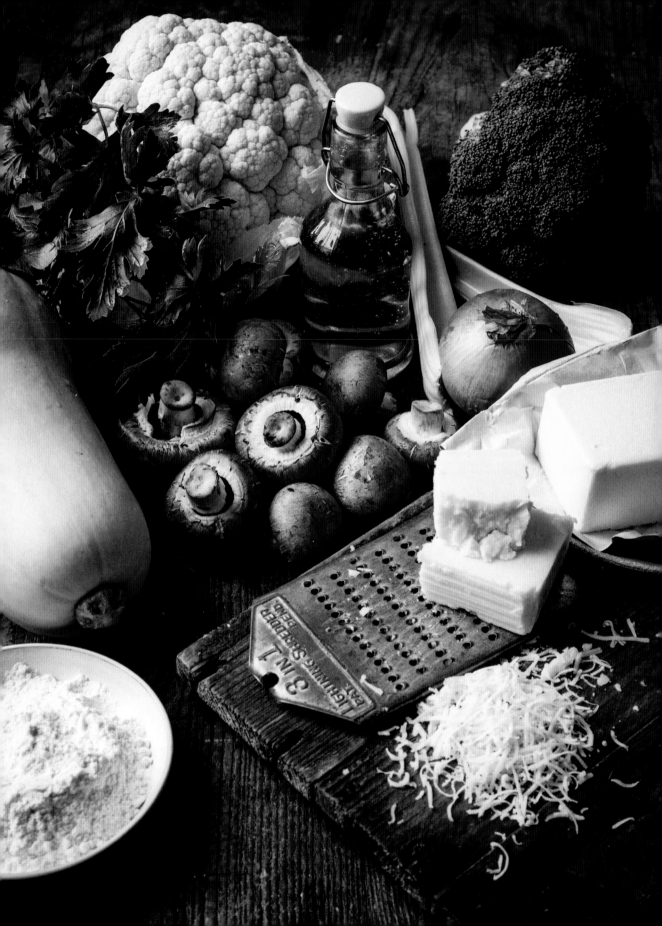

Spinach, ricotta and Parma ham lasagne

We've done quite a few lasagne recipes in our time and we're chuffed with this new one. It's rich, tasty and delicious, but not heavy, and it's easy to make, as we use frozen spinach, precooked lasagne sheets and a jar of tomato passata. It's an assembly job really and a cracking good dish.

Serves 4

500g frozen spinach, defrosted

200g ricotta

a few rasps of nutmeg

400ml passata

200ml single cream

small bunch of basil, finely chopped

2 garlic cloves, crushed

1/4 tsp cinnamon

1 tsp dried oregano

9 lasagne sheets (the precooked kind)

8 slices of Parma ham

75g Parmesan cheese, grated

2 blocks of mozzarella (about 600g), torn apart

salt and black pepper

Preheat the oven to 200°C/Fan 180°C/Gas 6.

Squeeze out as much liquid from the spinach as you can, chop the spinach roughly and mix it with the ricotta. Season with nutmeg, salt and pepper.

Mix the passata with the cream, basil, garlic, cinnamon and oregano. Season with salt and pepper and mix thoroughly.

Spread a quarter of the passata mixture over the base of a rectangular oven dish, then place 3 sheets of lasagne over it. Take about a third of the spinach and ricotta mixture and drop it in teaspoonfuls over the lasagne. Tear up 4 of the slices of Parma ham and drape them in between the spinach. Sprinkle over some Parmesan and mozzarella and top with another quarter of the passata mixture. Cover with 3 sheets of lasagne and repeat the spinach, Parma ham, Parmesan and mozzarella, and passata layers. Add a final 3 sheets of lasagne, then the last of the spinach and the passata. Top with the remaining mozzarella and grated Parmesan.

Bake in the oven for 30 minutes until brown and bubbling. Leave to stand for 10 minutes before serving.

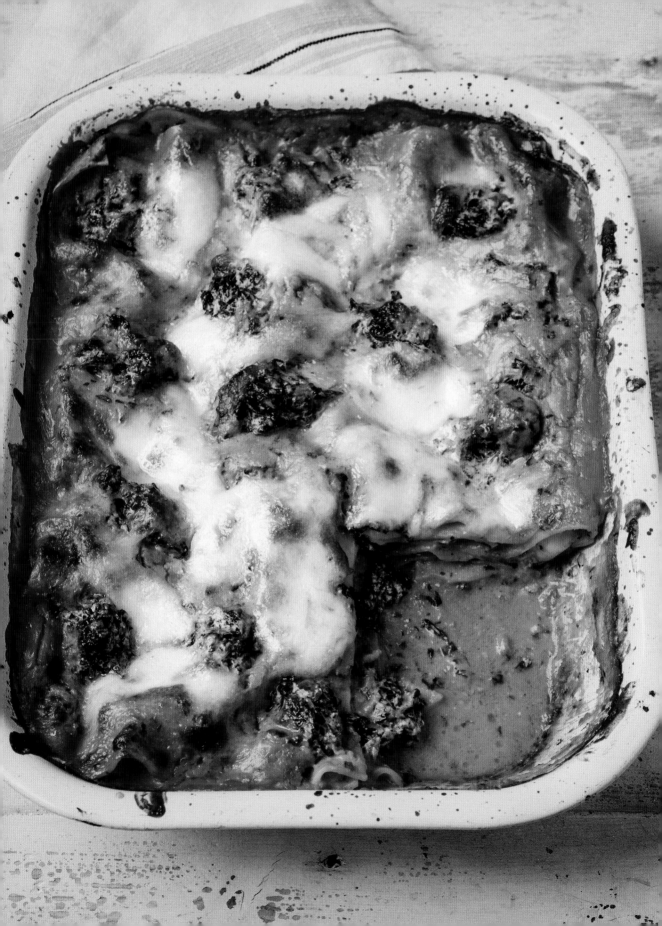

Coq au vin cobbler

We've done recipes for classic coq au vin – or as we like to call it 'love in a transit' – before, but for this book we decided to turn it into a cobbler. There's all that lovely French flavour with a crunchy topping. The cobbles are like savoury scones and give you a hearty carbohydrate treat – delicious mashed into the gravy.

Serves 4

2 tbsp olive oil

12 button onions or shallots, peeled

50g bacon lardons

2 tbsp plain flour

1 tsp rubbed sage

4 skinless, boneless chicken thighs, diced

2 skinless, boneless chicken breasts, diced

150g button mushrooms, halved if large

500ml red wine

200ml chicken stock

large thyme sprig

2 bay leaves

salt and black pepper

Cobbler topping

200g self-raising flour

1 tsp baking powder

small bunch of parsley, very finely chopped

1 egg

75ml buttermilk (see p.36)

First cook the filling. Heat the oil in a large flameproof casserole dish and add the onions or shallots. Cook until they're lightly coloured on all sides, then remove them from the dish and set aside.

Add the bacon lardons to the casserole dish and fry until they're crisp and some of the fat has rendered out. Remove and set aside.

Mix the flour with the rubbed sage and add plenty of salt and pepper. Toss the chicken and mushrooms in the flour, then fry them in the casserole dish until lightly browned – do this in a couple of batches if you like, so you don't overcrowd the pan. Pour in the red wine and bring to the boil, then reduce the heat and simmer until the wine has reduced by about two thirds. Add the stock, put the bacon and onions or shallots back in the dish and add the thyme and bay leaves.

Bring to the boil, then turn down the heat, cover with a lid, and simmer for 30 minutes until the onions or shallots are tender and the chicken is cooked through. Remove the lid and continue to simmer until the gravy is reduced – the consistency should be similar to single cream.

Preheat the oven to 200°C/Fan 180°C/Gas 6. While the chicken is cooking, make the cobbler topping. Mix the flour with the baking powder and plenty of salt. Stir in the parsley, followed by the egg and the buttermilk – you should end up with a slightly sticky dough. When the chicken is done, drop heaped tablespoons of this dough on top, then put the dish in the oven.

Bake for about 20 minutes until the cobbler topping is well risen and a rich golden brown. Leave it to sit for 5–10 minutes before serving.

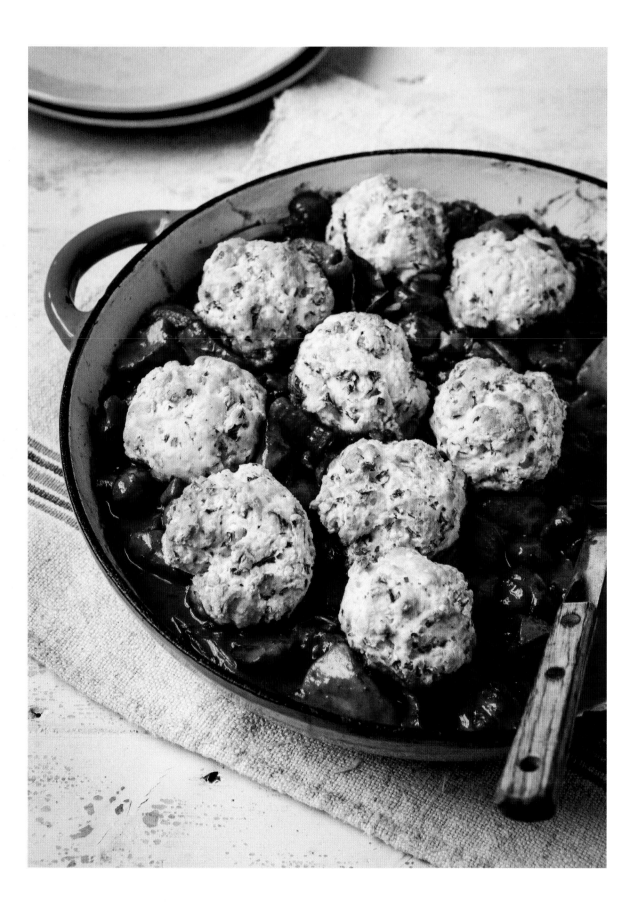

Chicken pie with a corn crust

With the corn and the chipotle paste, this chicken dish has a hint of the TexMex about it – and we love a bit of TexMex. The crust works brilliantly with the spicy chicken filling and this will keep the hungriest of cowboys and cowgirls happy!

Serves 4

1 tbsp olive oil

1 onion, finely chopped

1 red pepper, diced

1 green pepper, diced

3 garlic cloves, finely chopped

1 tsp ground cumin

½ tsp cinnamon

½ tsp allspice

¼ tsp cloves

1 tbsp chipotle paste

large thyme sprig

2 bay leaves

400g boneless chicken thighs, diced

200g butternut squash, diced

200ml chicken stock

250ml passata

salt and black pepper

Crust

500g sweetcorn kernels, defrosted if frozen

50g butter

1 tbsp fine cornmeal or plain flour

1 tsp baking powder

75g Cheddar cheese, grated

a few knobs of butter

Heat the oil in a large flameproof casserole dish. Add the onion and peppers and cook for a few minutes until they're starting to soften, then add the garlic, spices and chipotle paste. Cook for another couple of minutes, then add the herbs, chicken and butternut squash. Stir to coat all the chicken with the spices and season with plenty of salt and pepper.

Add the chicken stock and passata. Bring to the boil, then turn down the heat and partially cover the dish. Cook until the sauce has reduced down and the vegetables are tender.

Preheat the oven to 200°C/Fan 180°C/Gas 6. For the corn crust, put half the sweetcorn in a food processor and blitz it until smooth. Add the butter, cornmeal or flour, the baking powder and plenty of seasoning and blitz again to combine. Finally, add the rest of the sweetcorn and process briefly so the mixture keeps some texture. It should have a dropping consistency.

Stir a third of the cheese into the corn mix, then spoon this over the chicken. Sprinkle with the rest of the cheese and dot with butter. Bake in the oven for 30 minutes until the crust is golden brown and the filling is bubbling.

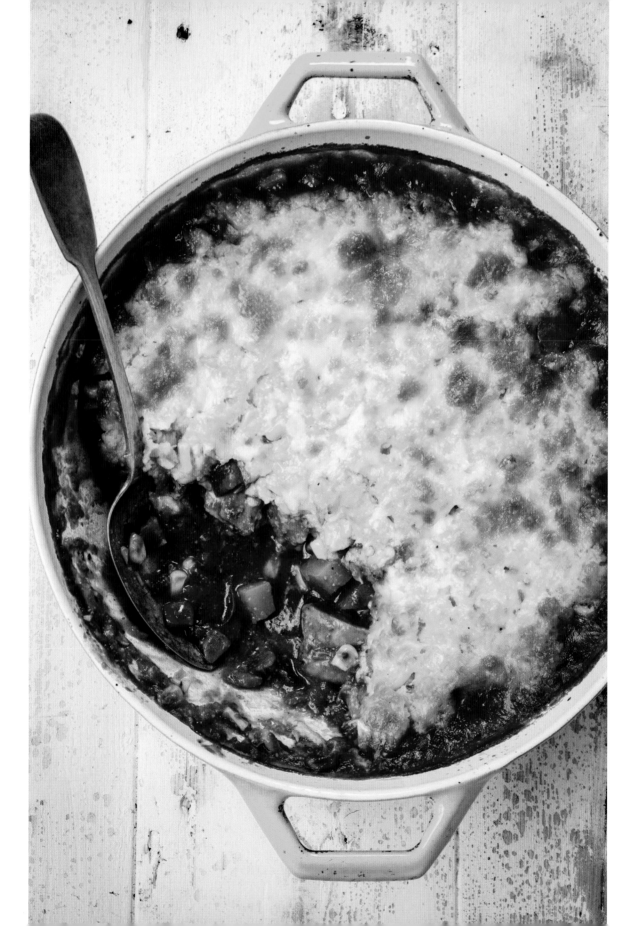

Pot-roast chicken

Everyone loves a roast chicken but it can be a bit of a palaver – and involves lots of pots and pans. With a pot-roast, the vegetables, gravy and bird are all cooked together and the veg get loads of lovely chickeny flavour. This is a proper Sunday lunch without the hassle.

Serves 4–6

1 tbsp olive oil

15g butter

100g bacon lardons

150g baby new potatoes, left whole

2 carrots, cut into chunks

2 celery sticks, cut into chunks

200g button mushrooms, left whole

1 chicken

2 bouquet garnis (tarragon, bay, thyme and parsley)

2 strips of pared lemon zest

1 garlic bulb, split into cloves but not peeled

100ml white wine

250ml chicken stock

2 or 3 leeks, cut into chunks

salt and black pepper

To serve

1 tbsp finely chopped tarragon leaves

1 tbsp finely chopped parsley leaves

Preheat the oven to 200°C/Fan 180°C/Gas 6. Heat the oil and butter in a large flameproof casserole dish, then add the bacon, potatoes, carrots and celery. Cook over a medium to high heat until everything is well browned, the bacon looks crisp and plenty of fat has rendered out. Add the mushrooms when everything else is nearly ready. Remove the vegetables and bacon with a slotted spoon and set them aside.

Take the chicken and put one bouquet garni and the lemon zest in the cavity. Place the chicken in the casserole dish, breast down, and brown it well on all sides, then leave it breast-side up. Sprinkle the garlic around the chicken and tuck in the other bouquet garni. Arrange all the browned vegetables and bacon around the sides, then season well.

Pour the wine around the chicken and bring it to the boil. Allow it to boil for a couple of minutes, then add the stock. Turn the heat down and put a lid on the dish. Transfer it to the oven and leave to cook for 30 minutes, then add the leeks. Put the lid back on and put the dish back in the oven for another 15 minutes.

Take the lid off and leave the dish in the oven for another 15 minutes to allow the chicken to crisp up. Check that it is cooked through by piercing the fattest part of the thigh – the juices should run clear. The legs should also feel loose.

Transfer the chicken to a warm serving platter, draining off any liquid from the cavity back into the casserole dish. Using a slotted spoon, arrange the vegetables around the chicken. Cover with foil and leave the chicken to rest and keep warm.

Squash the garlic flesh out of the cloves back into the gravy. Put the casserole dish on the hob, bring the gravy to the boil and reduce by about half until it is nice and creamy. Strain it into a jug and stir in the tarragon and parsley.

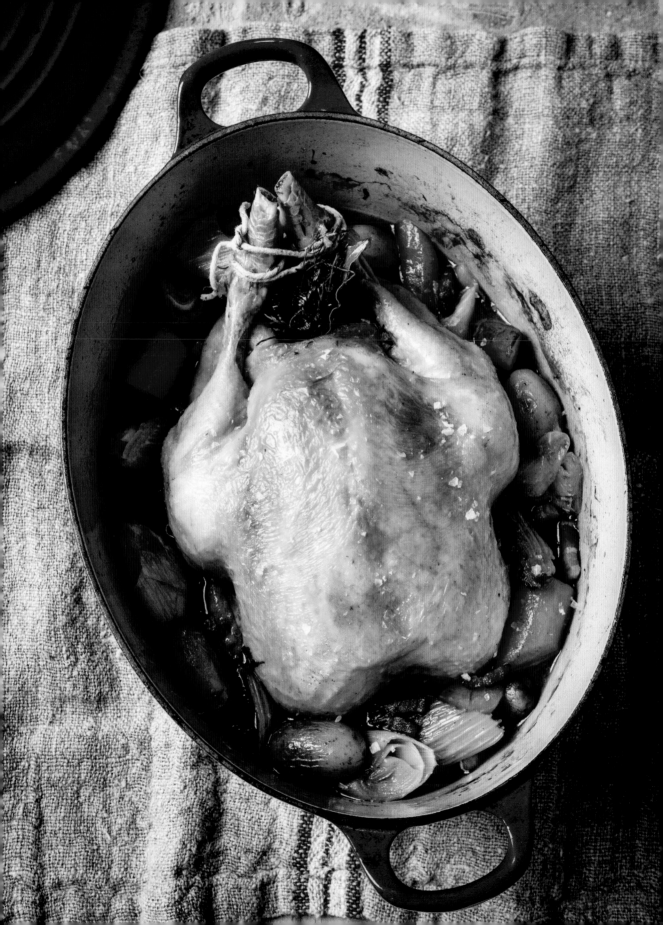

Chilli with nachos and cheese

We can't tell you how good this is – you just have to taste it. Yes, there are quite a few ingredients but a lot of them are spices and the prep is easy, just a bit of chopping. The nachos topping is amazing and you end up with different textures – crunchy on the top and softer at the bottom, with the juicy, spicy chilli underneath. Naughty but definitely nice.

Serves 4

2 tbsp olive oil
1 large onion, finely diced
2 celery sticks diced
1 red pepper, diced
400g minced beef
200g minced pork
4 garlic cloves, finely chopped
1 tbsp dried oregano
1 tbsp ground cumin
1 tsp chilli powder
1 tsp ground cinnamon
1 tsp ground coriander
1 tbsp light soft brown sugar
400g can of tomatoes
2 x 400g cans of red kidney
    beans, drained and rinsed
400ml beef stock or water
30g dark chocolate
salt and black pepper

Topping
200g tortilla chips
200g Cheddar cheese, grated

To serve
soured cream
fresh coriander leaves
lime wedges

Heat the oil in a large flameproof casserole dish. Add the onion, celery and red pepper and cook over a low heat until the onion has softened and turned translucent. Turn up the heat and add the meat. Leave it for a minute to brown on the underside, then start breaking it up with a spoon and turning it until it's all completely browned. Reduce the heat.

Add the garlic, oregano, spices and sugar and season with salt and pepper. Stir for a couple of minutes, then add the tomatoes, kidney beans and stock. Bring to the boil, cover and turn down the heat. Leave the chilli to simmer for an hour, stirring regularly to make sure it isn't catching on the bottom of the pan. Remove the lid, add the chocolate and stir until it has melted.

Preheat the oven to 200°C/Fan 180°C/Gas 6, or heat your grill to its highest setting. Meanwhile, continue to cook the chilli for another 15 minutes, until the sauce is very thick and well reduced – you don't want to put the nachos on to a liquid mixture.

Arrange the tortilla chips over the chilli and top with the cheese. Grill or bake them for at least 10 minutes until the cheese has melted and started to brown. Serve immediately with soured cream, some coriander leaves and lime wedges.

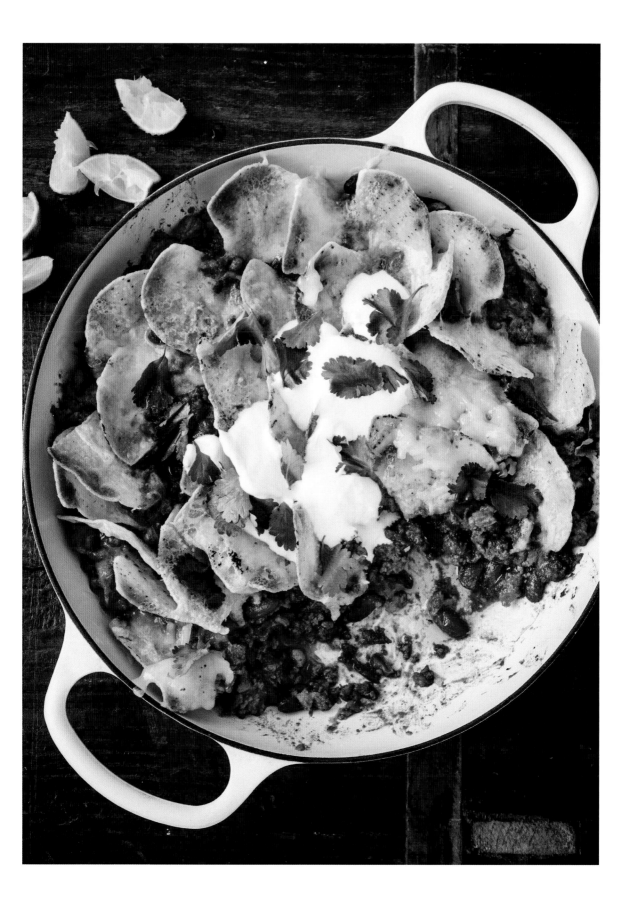

Special shepherd's pie

We weren't sure at first that we could make a shepherd's pie into a one pot, but magicians that we are we found a way – a nice sliced potato topping that doesn't need to be precooked. Don't worry if there looks like quite a lot of liquid when you first take the pie out of the oven. Be patient and let it be for 10 minutes – the potatoes will absorb the tasty juices perfectly and they'll be all sticky and delicious.

Serves 4

1 tbsp olive oil

500g minced or finely diced lamb

1 large onion, finely diced

2 carrots, finely diced

2 celery sticks, finely diced

2 garlic cloves, finely chopped

1 large rosemary sprig, leaves finely chopped

1 tsp dried oregano

½ tsp cinnamon

150ml red wine

200g canned tomatoes

300ml lamb stock

2 tsp anchovy sauce (optional)

salt and black pepper

Topping

600g floury potatoes, washed but unpeeled

100g Cheddar cheese, grated

Heat the oil in a large flameproof casserole dish. Add half the meat, press it down on to the base of the dish and leave it to develop a crust, then turn it and break it up. When the meat is well seared all over, remove it and set it aside, then repeat with the second batch. Remove and set that aside, then spoon off most of the fat that will have accumulated in the bottom of the dish.

Add the onion, carrots and celery. Cook them over a medium heat for up to 10 minutes, until they are softening and just starting to take on some colour, then add the garlic and cook for another couple of minutes. Put the meat back in the dish and add the herbs and cinnamon.

Turn up the heat and pour in the red wine. Bring it to the boil and allow the wine to reduce by half, then add the tomatoes, stock and anchovy sauce, if using. Season with salt and pepper. Bring to the boil again, then turn down and simmer, partially covered with a lid, for about 15 minutes. The sauce should reduce down a little in this time, but it mustn't get too dry – some of the liquid is necessary to help cook the potatoes. Preheat the oven to 200°C/Fan 180°C/Gas 6.

While the filling is cooking, prepare the potatoes. Slice them as thinly as you can, preferably with a mandolin, as this will give the most even results. Don't rinse the slices. Arrange the potatoes, one layer at a time, over the meat sauce, seasoning each layer with salt and pepper and sprinkling in a little of the cheese. Press the potatoes down with the flat of your hands – some of the liquid from the sauce should momentarily submerge them. Top with the rest of the cheese.

Put the lid on and bake in the oven for 30 minutes, by which time the potatoes should be close to knife tender. Then take the lid off and bake for another 30 minutes, until the cheese is brown and bubbling and the potatoes are done. Leave the pie to stand for 5–10 minutes before serving. The potatoes will absorb any excess liquid and the potatoes will be infused with the flavour of the meat.

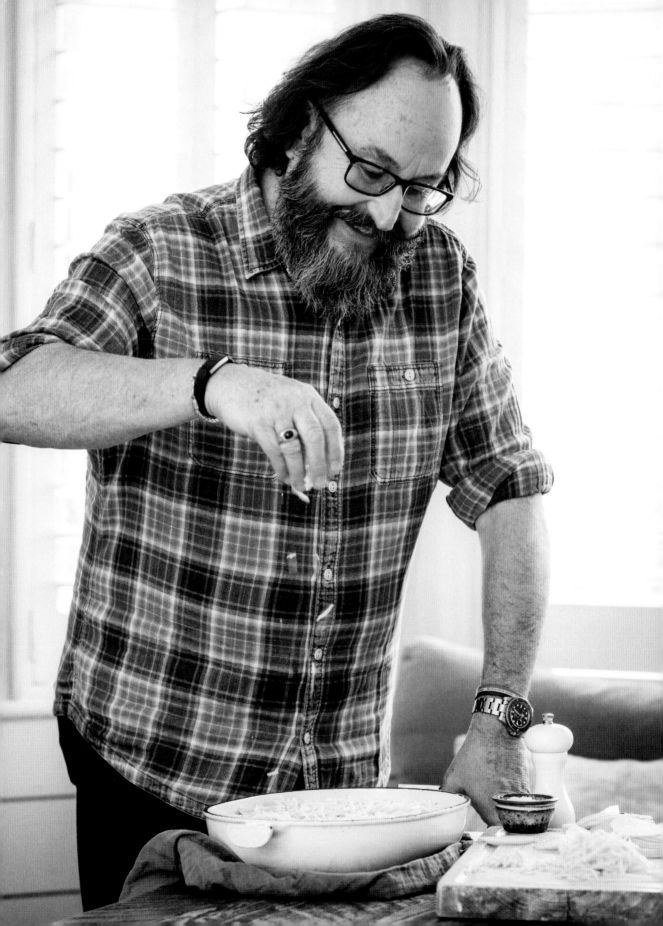

Steak and mushroom pie

No Hairy Biker book would be complete without a pie or two, and ready-rolled puff pastry makes it easy to bake a one pot pie. We do recommend adding the oysters or mussels. They are a traditional ingredient in steak pies and they add a nice smoky flavour.

Serves 4

1 x 320g ready-rolled puff pastry sheet

750g braising steak, diced

50g plain flour

3 tbsp olive oil

300g chestnut mushrooms, halved

1 large onion, finely chopped

3 garlic cloves, chopped

1 large thyme sprig

2 bay leaves

300ml red wine

300ml beef stock

1 tsp Worcestershire sauce

½ tsp Dijon mustard

1 can of smoked mussels or oysters (optional)

1 egg, beaten with 1 tbsp water

salt and black pepper

Unroll the pastry and cut a round or rectangle that will fit snugly into your casserole dish or pan. Lay it on a piece of greaseproof paper and put it in the fridge to chill. If you're feeling artistic, use the scraps to cut out decorations for the top of the pie.

Season the steak with salt and pepper and dust it with the flour. Pat off any excess. Heat a tablespoon of the oil in a large flameproof casserole dish or pan and fry the steak until browned. It's best to do this in a couple of batches so you don't overcrowd the dish. Remove the browned meat and set it aside, then add the remaining oil and briskly fry the mushrooms. When they're brown, remove them and set aside, then add the onion. Turn down the heat and cook the onion until soft, then stir in the garlic and cook for another couple of minutes.

Put the beef back in the dish or pan and add the thyme and bay leaves. Turn up the heat and pour in the red wine. Leave it to bubble for a few minutes, then add the beef stock, Worcestershire sauce and mustard – the steak should be just about covered. Season with salt and pepper.

Bring to the boil, then turn down the heat to a simmer and put the lid on the dish or cover tightly with foil. Leave to simmer for an hour and a half, checking regularly to make sure the mixture isn't sticking. Add the cooked mushrooms and continue to simmer for another 30 minutes or until the beef is tender. Remove the lid and simmer to reduce the liquid – it needs to be the consistency of gravy. Set the dish aside so the beef can cool down.

When you want to cook the pie, preheat the oven to 200°C/Fan 180°C/Gas 6. Roughly chop the mussels or oysters, if using, and scatter these on top of the beef. Lay the pastry over the top and add any decoration, then brush with beaten egg. Cut a couple of slits in the centre of the pastry. Bake in the oven for 35–40 minutes until the pastry is a rich golden brown and well risen and the filling is piping hot and bubbling.

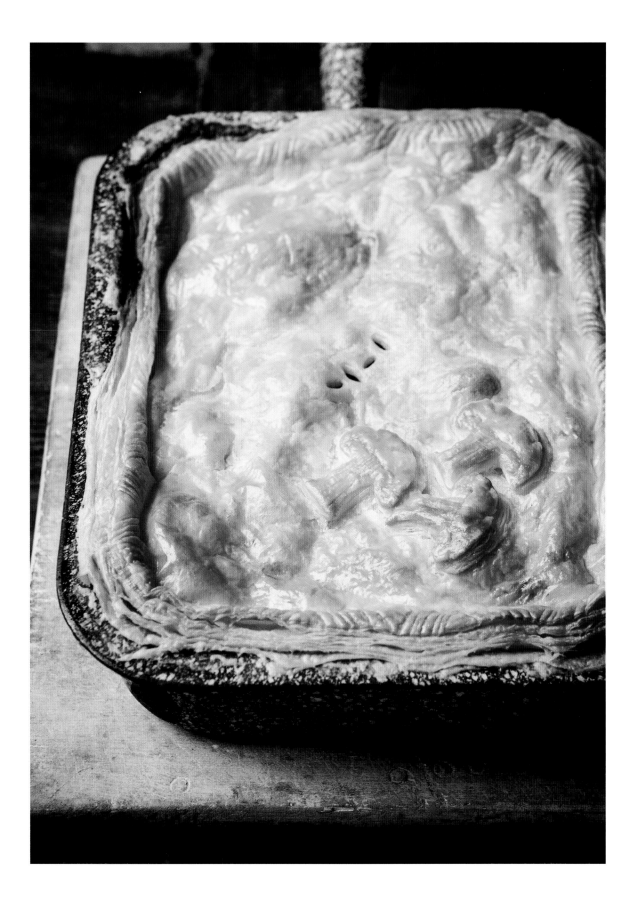

Pot-roast beef

This is the Sunday lunch we were both brought up on. Pot roasting is an excellent way of cooking a nice piece of silverside or topside and makes a cracking feast, with the best gravy imaginable. It does need to cook for a long time, but that gives you a chance to relax, read the papers and just enjoy the aromas from the oven. Great with Yorkshire pud – but oops, that would need another pot!

Serves 4

2 tbsp olive oil

12 shallots, peeled

2 celery sticks, roughly chopped

2 large carrots, cut into chunks

400g new potatoes, left whole or halved

2 tsp mustard powder

1kg silverside or beef topside, extra fat removed

4 garlic cloves, finely chopped

1 thyme sprig

2 bay leaves

150ml red wine

600ml beef stock

2 tsp butter

2 tsp plain flour

1–2 tsp redcurrant jelly

salt and black pepper

Preheat the oven to 160°C/Fan 140°C/Gas 3.

Heat the oil in a large flameproof casserole dish that has a lid. Add the shallots, celery, carrots and potatoes. Cook over a high heat until they're all starting to colour, then remove them from the dish and set aside.

Mix the mustard powder with salt and pepper, then dust the beef with the mixture. Add the beef to the casserole dish and sear it on all sides. Arrange the vegetables around the beef and add the garlic, thyme and bay leaves. Pour in the wine and bring to the boil. Leave it to bubble for a few minutes, then add the stock and bring to the boil again.

Put the lid on the dish and place it in the oven for 2 hours, turning it round halfway through the cooking time. Remove the dish from the oven and check the meat for doneness – it should be tender. Transfer the beef and vegetables to a warm platter and cover them loosely with foil.

Knead the butter and flour together to make a paste, then whisk this into the cooking liquid, a little at a time, until it thickens to a gravy. Taste for seasoning, then stir in the redcurrant jelly, again, a little at a time, to taste. Serve the gravy with the beef and vegetables.

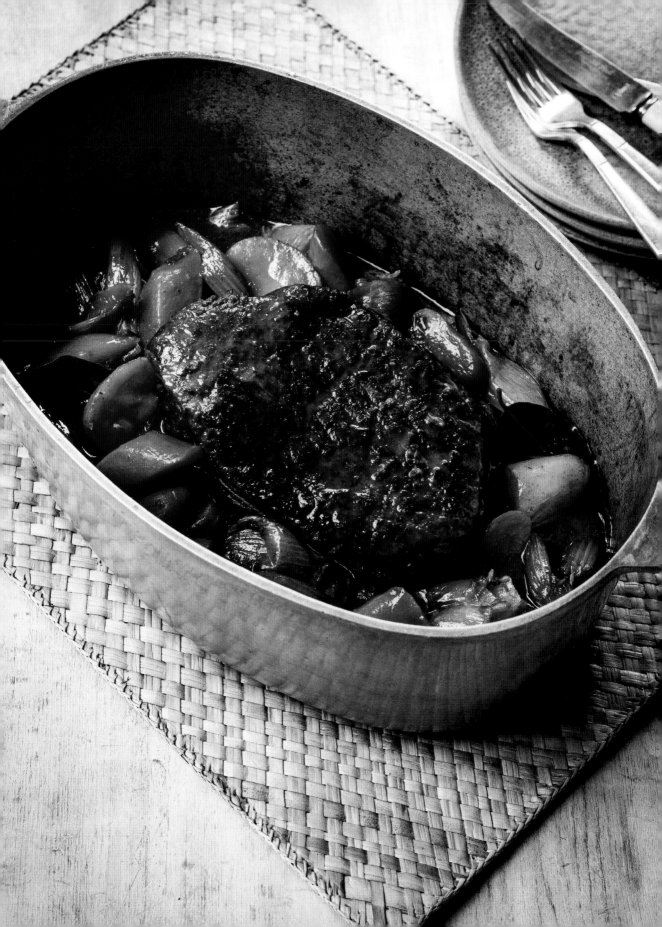

Turkey and ham Christmas casserole

This is a great way to use up any leftover turkey and ham at Christmas, or you can substitute chicken at any other time of year. The topping is made from stuffing ingredients and turns out beautifully crunchy and tasty – of course, many of us think the stuffing is the best part of Christmas dinner. A fab festive feast.

Serves 4

50g butter

3 leeks, cut into rounds

30g plain flour

100ml white wine

500ml chicken stock

100ml double cream

400g cooked turkey (or chicken), diced

150g ham, diced

2 tarragon sprigs, leaves finely chopped

100g peas, defrosted

6 cubes of frozen spinach, defrosted

salt and black pepper

Stuffing crust

100g breadcrumbs

1 small onion, grated

100g chestnuts, grated

50g dried cranberries, soaked in warm water (optional)

2 tsp dried sage

small bunch of parsley, finely chopped

large knob of butter

First make the filling. Heat the butter in a large flameproof casserole dish. When it has melted, add the leeks with plenty of seasoning and turn down the heat. Cover the dish with a lid and leave the leeks to cook gently until tender. Stir regularly and try not to let them take on any colour.

Stir the flour into the dish to form a roux around the leeks. Add the wine and stir vigorously – it will thicken considerably. Gradually add the stock, stirring constantly, until you have incorporated it all, then add the cream. Fold in the turkey or chicken, ham, tarragon and peas. Squeeze any excess water from the spinach, then stir the spinach into the dish. Taste for seasoning and add salt and pepper as needed.

To make the topping, mix the breadcrumbs, onion, chestnuts, drained cranberries and the herbs, then season with plenty of salt and pepper. Sprinkle this mixture over the top of the filling, then dot with butter. Bake in the oven for 25–30 minutes until the filling is bubbling and breaking through the crisp, golden-brown topping.

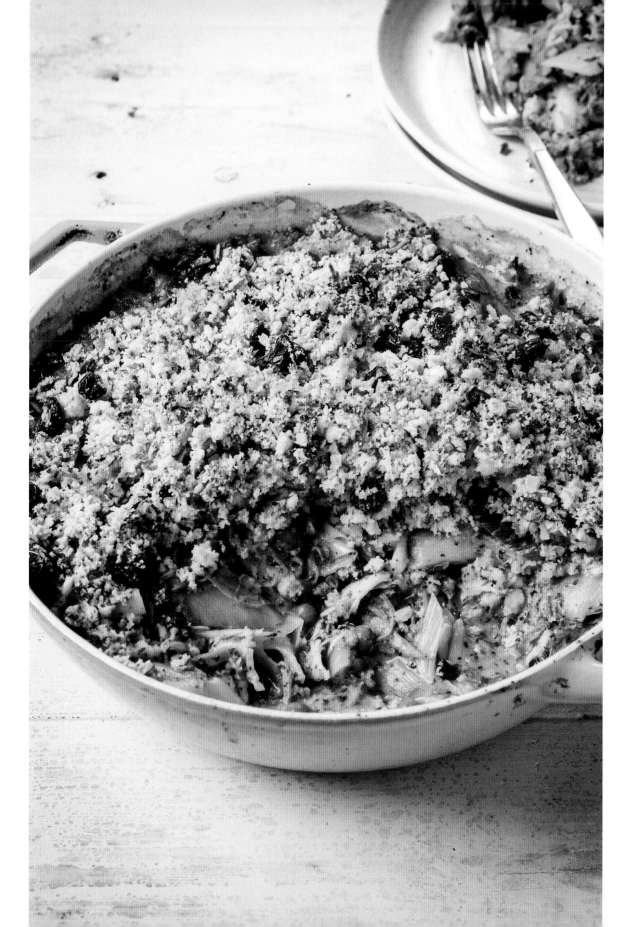

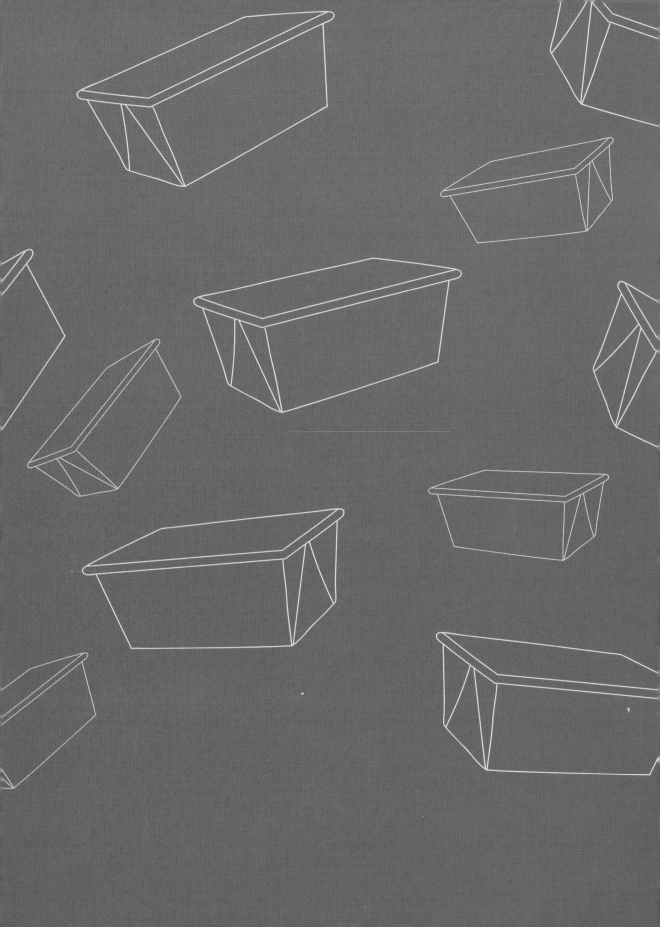

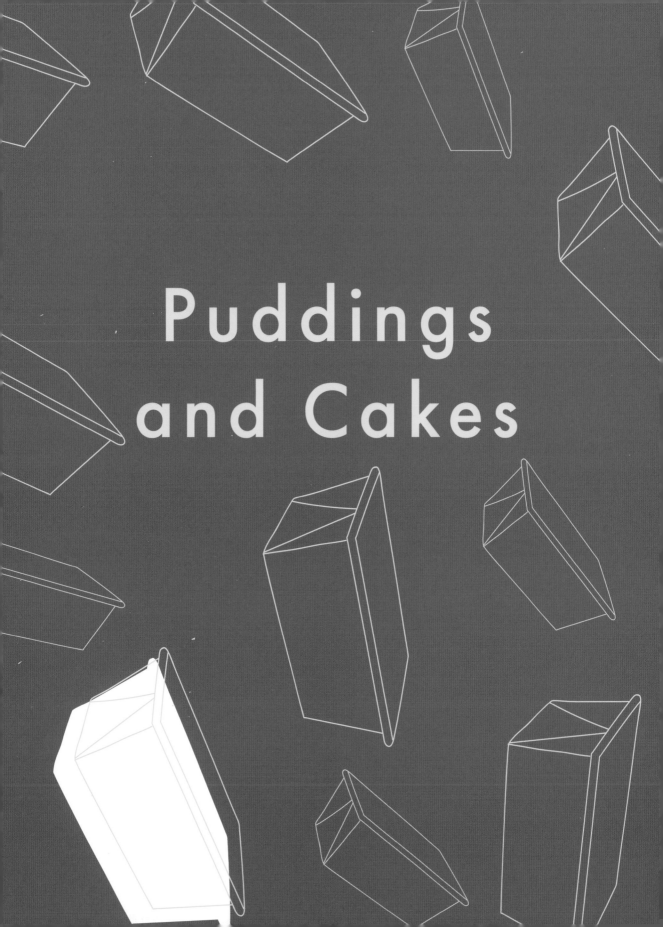

Puddings
and Cakes

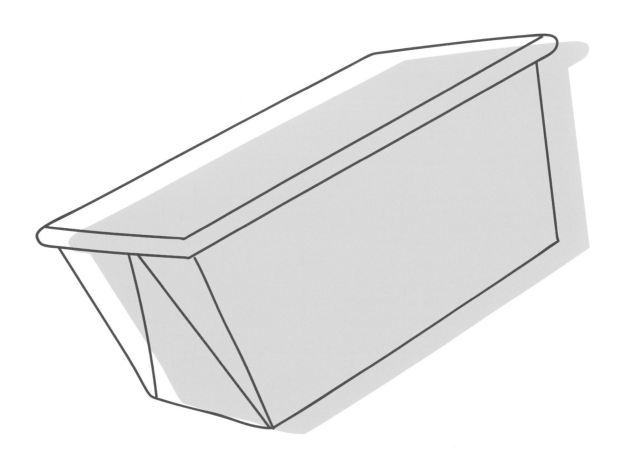

Anzac flapjacks

These yummy little delights are a beautiful marriage between coconutty Anzac biscuits, much-loved in Australia and New Zealand, and our good old British date flapjacks. They are very happy together and we think you will be too.

Makes about 12 squares

250g butter
250g light brown sugar
100g golden syrup
pinch of salt
100g desiccated coconut
400g porridge oats
200g dates, pitted and
    chopped

Preheat the oven to 160°C/Fan 140°C/Gas 3. Line a 30 x 20cm straight-sided baking tin with baking paper.

Put the butter, sugar and golden syrup into a large pan and melt them together. Add a generous pinch of salt, then stir in the coconut, oats and dates.

Pile the mixture into the baking tin and spread it evenly. Press it down as firmly as you can – this will help the mixture stick together.

Bake in the oven for 25 minutes for a chewy flapjack, another 5 minutes for a slightly crisper one. Make sure the top is turning golden brown before you remove the tin from the oven. The mixture will be soft, but don't worry, it will firm up as it cools.

Leave to cool for 10 minutes, then score into squares. Do not try to cut right through the flapjacks until they are completely cool, as they will break up. When they have cooled and are firm, cut into squares and store in an airtight tin.

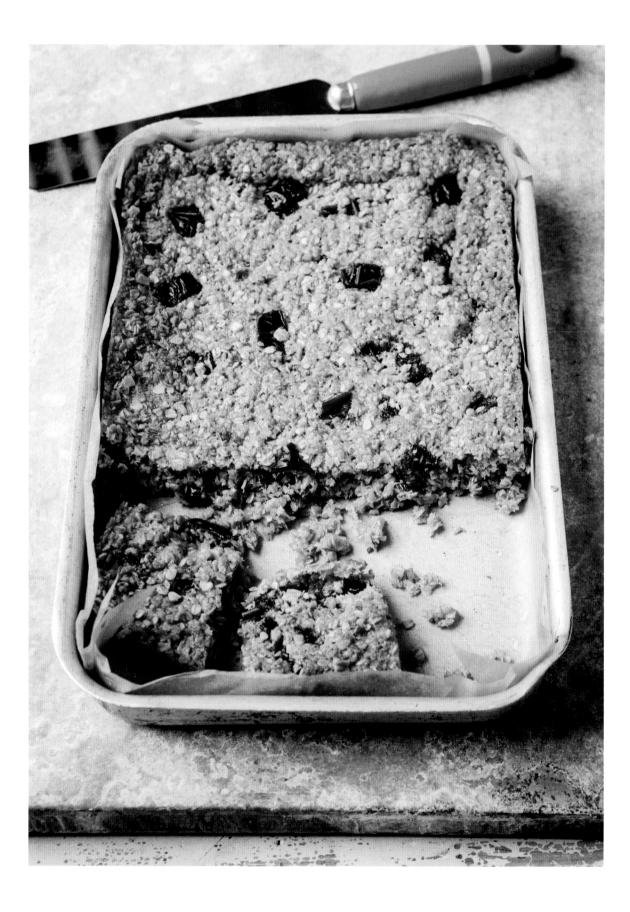

Chocolate brownies

We're always more than happy to experiment with brownie recipes and this one is made by a nice and easy all-in-one method that works well. Add the baking powder if you like a cakey brownie that rises slightly, but if you prefer a dense-textured brownie, leave it out. Either way these are the business – a tray bake classic.

Makes 16 squares

150g butter
225g granulated sugar
80g cocoa powder
pinch of salt
1 tsp vanilla extract
2 eggs
75g plain flour
½ tsp baking powder
(optional)
100g chocolate, chopped,
or chocolate chips
100g hazelnuts, halved
100g glacé cherries, rinsed
and dried

Preheat the oven to 170°C/Fan 150°C/Gas 3 ½. Line a 30 x 20cm tin with a large piece of baking paper, so it sticks up above the tin.

Put the butter, sugar and cocoa powder in a heatproof bowl and add a generous pinch of salt. Set the bowl over a pan of simmering water and let everything melt together, stirring regularly. The mixture will have quite a grainy texture but that's fine.

Remove the bowl from the pan and add the vanilla extract, then beat in the eggs, one at a time. Beat until the batter is glossy and smooth, then add the flour. Add the baking powder, if using, for a more cakey brownie.

Keep beating the mixture for a good minute – this is important for the final texture of the brownies. Add the chocolate, hazelnuts and cherries and stir them in. Scrape the batter into the prepared tin and smooth the top with a palette knife.

Bake in the oven for 20–25 minutes until the top looks dry and a skewer inserted into the centre comes out with moist crumbs attached to it. Lift the brownie out of the tin with the baking paper and transfer it to a rack. Leave it to cool before cutting into squares.

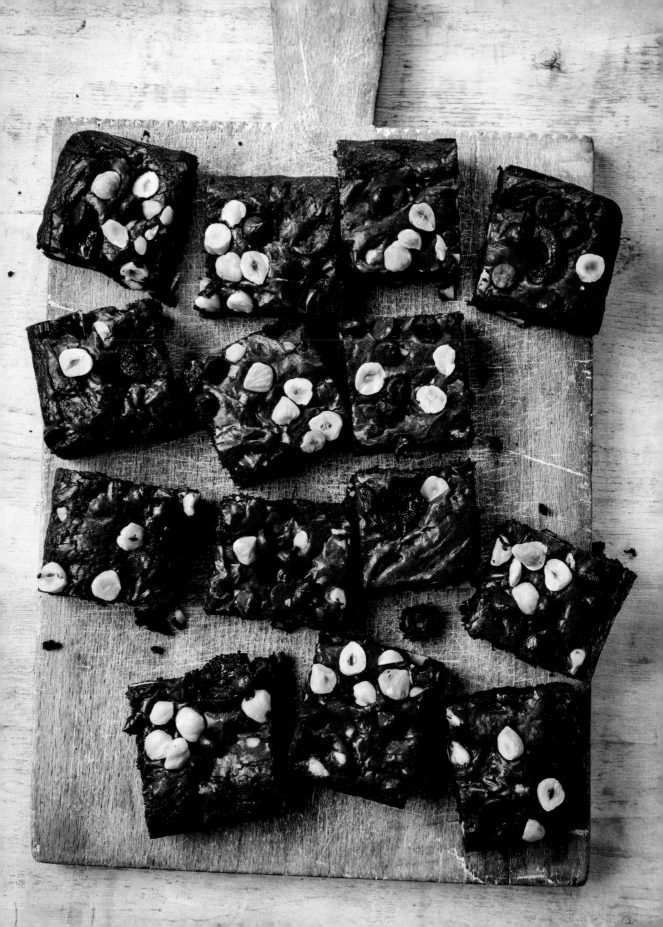

Bikers' rocky road!

Our new version of rocky road is quicker and cheaper than most, as it is all mixed in one bowl and made with cocoa powder instead of lots of chocolate. We've made it in a square tin, but you can also turn the mixture out on to cling film, roll it into a sausage shape and call it chocolate salami. Mega good either way.

Makes 9 squares or 18 triangles

150g caster sugar

4 egg yolks

175g butter, softened

100g cocoa powder

pinch of salt

50g raisins

50g glacé cherries, halved

50g soft dates, chopped

100g almonds, chopped

200g biscuits, such as digestive or shortbread, chopped into ½-1cm squares

25g small marshmallows (optional)

Note that this recipe does contain raw eggs, so make sure you buy eggs that are produced under the British Lion Code of Practice.

Put the sugar and egg yolks into a bowl and beat with a wooden spoon – don't whisk, as you don't want the mixture aerated. Add the butter and cocoa powder with a good pinch of salt and continue to beat until everything is well combined and you have a thick paste with a spreadable consistency.

Add the dried fruit, nuts and biscuits and stir well so they are as evenly distributed as possible throughout the mixture. Line a small baking tin, about 20 x 20cm, with cling film and spread the chocolate mixture evenly over it. Press in the marshmallows, if using.

Put the tin in the fridge for several hours, preferably overnight. To serve, slice into squares or triangles.

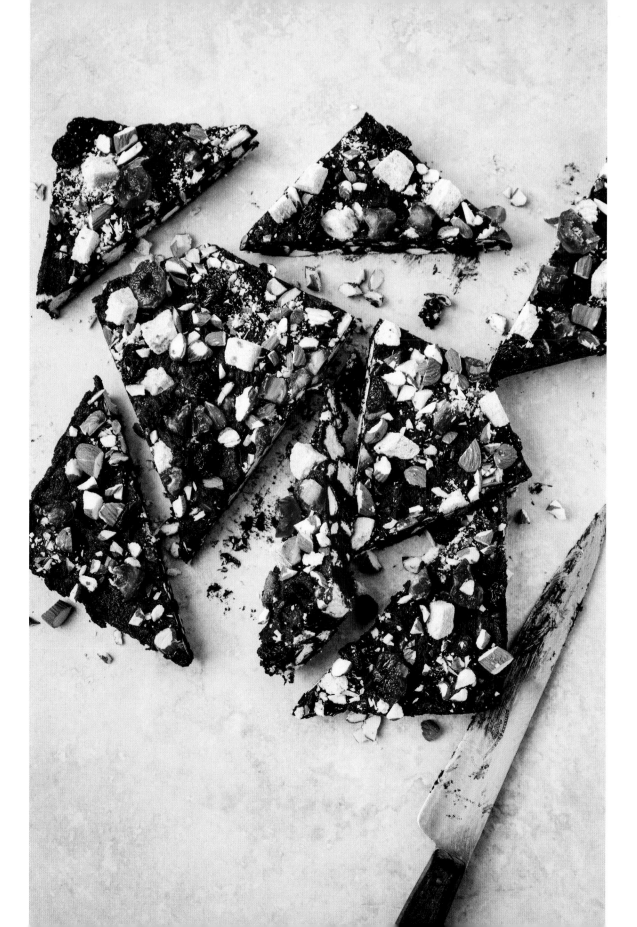

Belting banana bread

When bananas go a bit mottled and mushy, don't throw them away – they're just right for making some banana bread. This takes minutes to mix and uses mostly store-cupboard ingredients. Use your loaf and make this, then enjoy a slice with a nice cup of tea.

Makes 1 loaf

100g raisins
3 large ripe bananas
125ml vegetable oil
150g light soft brown sugar
pinch of salt
2 eggs
175g plain flour
1 tbsp mixed spice
2 tsp baking powder
½ tsp bicarbonate of soda

Preheat the oven to 180°C/Fan 160°C/Gas 4. Line a large (900g) loaf tin with baking paper.

Put the raisins in a large bowl and pour boiling water over them to help plump them up, then leave them to soak for 5 minutes. Drain, discard the soaking water and set the raisins aside.

Add the bananas to the bowl and mash them well. Add the vegetable oil and sugar and whisk until everything is well combined, then add a generous pinch of salt. Beat in the eggs, one at a time, then sprinkle in the flour, mixed spice, baking powder and bicarbonate of soda. Fold the wet and dry ingredients together carefully, then stir in the raisins.

Spoon the batter into the tin and bake for about an hour until the loaf is well risen and slightly cracked. A skewer should come out clean.

Leave the banana bread to cool in the tin and then store in an airtight container. This is good just as it is or toasted with butter.

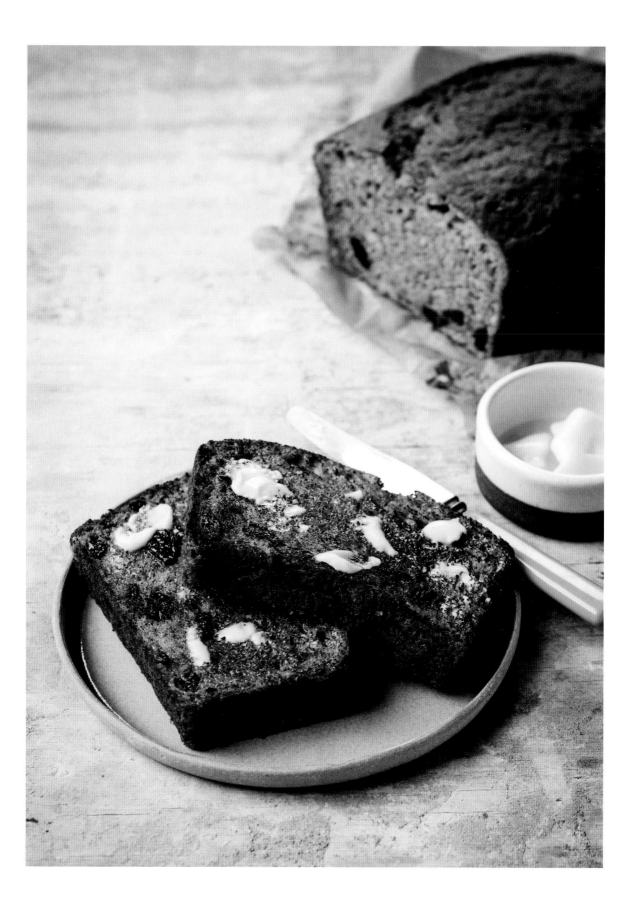

Giant cookie

This takes the biscuit! Even we couldn't scoff a cookie this big, but it looks spectacular and cuts nicely into 12 more modest wedges. Of course, you could bake the cookie dough as a rectangle or as individual cookies but that wouldn't be half as much fun.

Makes 12 slices

125g butter

100g soft light brown sugar

100g granulated sugar

125g peanut butter

1 egg

1 tsp vanilla extract

175g plain flour

pinch of bicarbonate of soda

pinch of baking powder

pinch of salt

75g salted roasted peanuts, ground to coarse crumbs

100g dried cherries, soaked in warm water and dried

100g fudge pieces or chocolate chips (optional)

Preheat the oven to 170°C/Fan 150°C/Gas 3 ½. Cut a round of baking paper, about 32cm in diameter, and place it on a 32cm pizza tray or a nice wide baking tray.

Using an electric hand whisk, beat the butter and sugars together until very light and fluffy. Beat in the peanut butter, followed by the egg and vanilla extract. Add the flour, bicarb and baking powder and a pinch of salt, then mix to a soft, thick dough. Fold in the ground salted peanuts, dried cherries and fudge pieces or chocolate chips, if using.

Put the dough in the centre of the baking paper and press it out to fill the circle, making sure you leave at least a centimetre border all the way round. Spread the dough as evenly as possible, preferably keeping the edges the same height as the centre.

Bake the cookie in the preheated oven for 18–20 minutes until it's lightly browned and slightly puffed up. It won't look completely cooked in the middle. This timing gives a fairly soft and chewy cookie, but if you want something crisper, bake for up to another 5 minutes.

Leave the cookie to cool for 5 minutes, then use a pizza wheel or a sharp knife to cut it into slices. Allow to cool completely, then eat or transfer the slices to an airtight tin.

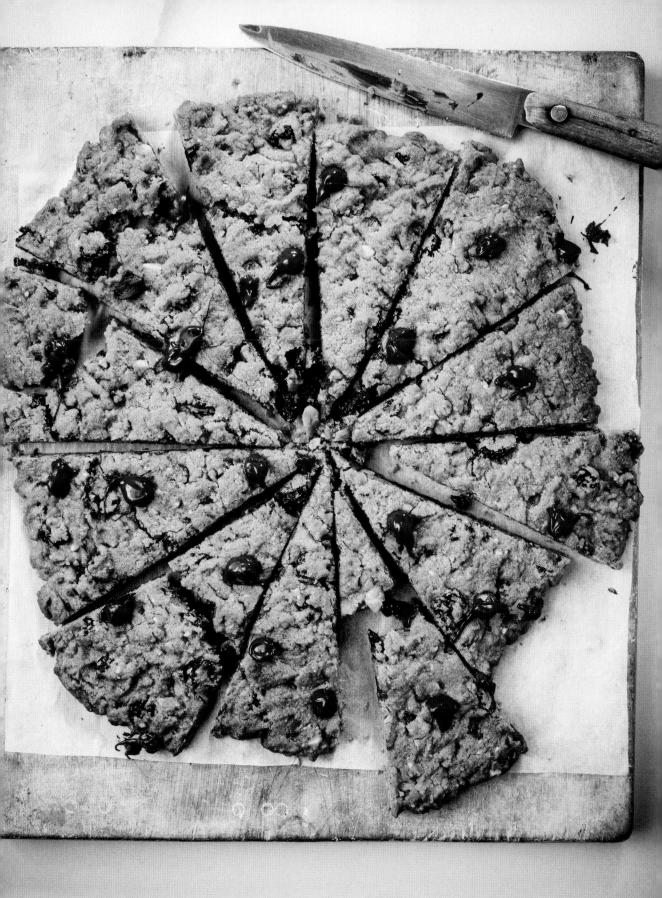

Spicy fruit loaf

There's only one problem with this excellent fruit loaf – it's best kept for a couple of days to mature before eating, and that's hard if you've smelt the aroma as it bakes in the oven. Ah well, do your best. We've suggested our fave fruit combo but feel free to vary or just use 400g mixed dried fruit.

Makes 1 loaf

150g sultanas or raisins

100g currants

100g glacé cherries, halved

50g prunes

350ml hot strong tea

2 balls of stem ginger, finely chopped (optional)

100g light soft brown sugar

2 eggs, beaten

300g wholemeal or white self-raising flour

2 tsp mixed spice

pinch of salt

Put all the dried fruit into a large bowl and pour over the tea – there should be enough to completely submerge the fruit. Cover and leave to soak for several hours, or preferably overnight. The fruit will swell up and the liquid will have thickened to a syrup.

When you are ready to bake the loaf, preheat the oven to 160°C/Fan 140°C/ Gas 3 and line a large (900g) loaf tin with baking paper.

Stir in the stem ginger, if using, into the fruit, followed by the sugar and the eggs. Sprinkle over the flour with the mixed spice and a generous pinch of salt, then stir everything together – the mixture should have a slow dropping consistency.

Pour the mixture into the prepared tin and bake for 60–75 minutes. Start checking after an hour – the loaf should have shrunk away from the sides and will be firm but springy when you press it. Leave it to cool in the tin.

Remove the loaf from the tin once cool, wrap it in cling film and leave it for a day or so before eating it, if possible. The top will become slightly glossy and sticky in that time. This keeps well in an airtight container for up to 2 weeks.

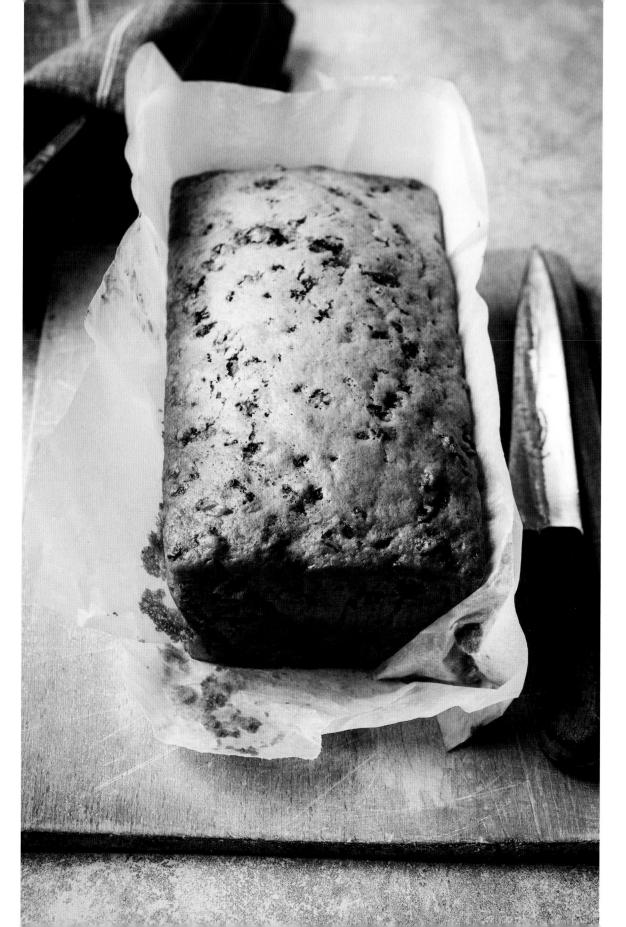

Apple streusel tray bake

Tray bakes are so quick and simple to make, even if you're not a Bake Off star. This one is a great invention, with its crunchy streusel topping, so give it a go.

Makes 12 squares

Streusel topping

100g plain flour

50g cold butter, diced

75g demerara sugar

½ tsp cinnamon

50g chopped walnuts

Cake

225g butter, softened

225g light brown sugar

300g self-raising flour

75g walnuts, chopped

2 tsp baking powder

1 tsp ground cinnamon

¼ tsp cloves

¼ tsp ground allspice

4 eggs

1–2 tbsp milk

large pinch of salt

Apples

4 eating apples, peeled and diced

2 tbsp demerara sugar

1 tsp ground cinnamon

Preheat the oven to 180°C/Fan 160°C/Gas 4. Line a 30 x 20cm baking tin with baking paper.

First make the streusel topping. Put the flour into a bowl with the butter, 50g of the sugar and the cinnamon. Rub the butter into the flour, then stir in the walnuts. Put the mixture in the fridge until you are ready to bake the cake.

Mix all the cake ingredients together with an electric hand whisk or in a food processor to form a smooth batter. Mix the diced apples with the sugar and cinnamon and fold them into the cake batter. Spoon the mixture into the baking tin and smooth it down.

Sprinkle the chilled streusel topping evenly over the batter, then sprinkle over the remaining sugar. Bake in the oven for 35–40 minutes until the cake is well risen and springy to touch. Leave it to cool in the tin for 10 minutes, then remove and place on a wire rack to cool completely. Cut into squares to serve.

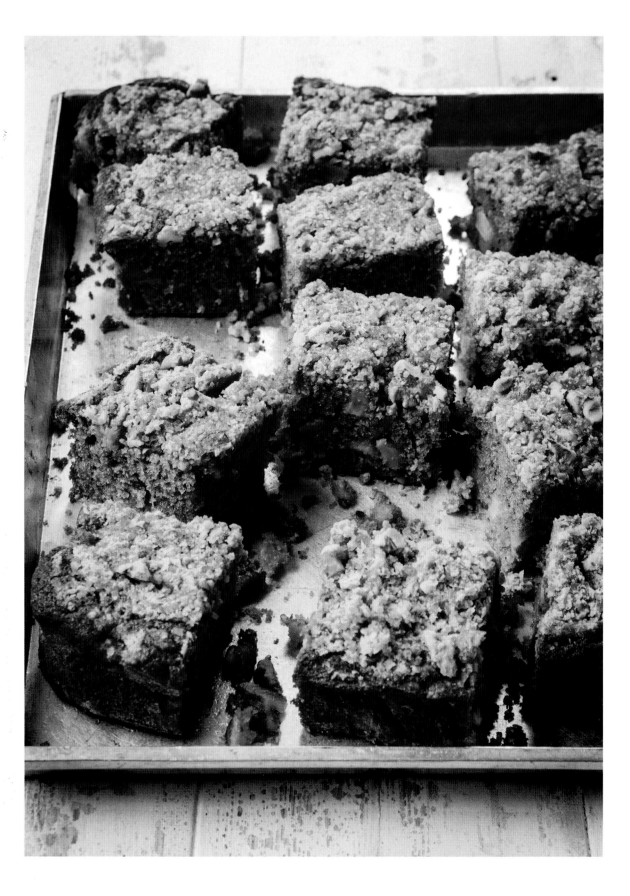

Peach tarte tatin

There's a savoury tarte tatin on page 134, but we wanted to include a luscious sweet version too. Once you've got the knack these are really easy to make. The peaches shouldn't be too ripe – they are cooked in the caramel and if they are too ripe they will just go mushy.

Serves 4

100g caster sugar

juice of 1 lemon

60g cold butter, diced

1–2 tsp rosewater (optional)

1 tsp cinnamon

5–6 firm peaches, peeled if you like, cut into wedges

1 x 320g all-butter puff pastry sheet

To serve
crème fraiche

Put the sugar and lemon juice in an ovenproof frying pan (preferably cast iron). Place the pan over a medium heat and leave the sugar to melt to a light golden caramel. Remove the pan from the heat and whisk in the butter. Stir in the rose water, if using, and the cinnamon.

Arrange the peach wedges over the caramel, then place the pan over a gentle heat and simmer for up to 10 minutes. Turn the peaches every so often until they are cooked through and the caramel is thick and syrupy.

If, when your peaches are cooked, the caramel is still very liquid, remove the peaches and continue to simmer the caramel until it has reduced and thickened. Put the peaches back in the pan and leave to cool completely.

Preheat the oven to 200°C/Fan 180°C/Gas 6. Roll out the pastry to about ½ cm thick, then cut out a round slightly bigger than your pan. Place the pastry over the peaches and tuck in the edges around the sides. Cut a few slits in the pastry to let steam escape.

Bake the tarte tatin in the oven for about 30 minutes – the pastry should be golden brown and you should be able to see the caramel sauce bubbling away underneath.

Remove the pan from the oven and leave to stand for 5 minutes to allow the sauce to thicken up a little – no longer or it will become too sticky to turn out properly. Very carefully turn the tart out on to a plate. Dislodge any reluctant peach wedges if there are any, and scrape out any sauce, then serve immediately with dollops of crème fraiche.

Blondies

Si: Dave's got his brownies but these little wonders are for me. Some say blondes have more fun, so give this recipe a go. Up the blondes, I say!

Makes 16 squares

175g butter
225g light soft brown sugar
pinch of salt
2 eggs
1 tsp vanilla extract
225g plain flour
½ tsp baking powder
150g white chocolate, broken into chunks
16 raspberries (optional)

Preheat the oven to 200°C/Fan 180°C/Gas 6. Line a 20cm square tin with baking paper.

Put the butter in a large bowl and set it over a pan of simmering water. When the butter has melted, remove the bowl from the heat and leave to cool for a few minutes. Whisk in the sugar with a pinch of salt, then add the eggs and vanilla extract. Fold in the flour, baking powder and white chocolate chunks.

Scrape the mixture into the prepared tin, then arrange the raspberries, if using, over the top, pressing them in lightly. Imagine you are putting them in the centre of each square.

Bake for about 25 minutes, until lightly coloured and just set on top. Remove from the oven, leave to cool in the tin and then cut into 16 small squares.

Rhubarb and orange crumble

Fruit crumbles never go out of fashion and rhubarb is probably our very favourite. The touch of orange brings out the flavour of the rhubarb and adds a tangy freshness. A simple classic, this is loved by all. Great with custard (see page 277 if you want to make your own).

Serves 4–6

butter, for greasing
500g rhubarb
1 large orange
100g light soft brown sugar

Topping

150g plain flour
½ tsp cinnamon
100g butter, softened, plus
   extra for dotting on the top
75g light soft brown sugar
75g porridge oats
pinch of salt

Preheat the oven to 180°C/Fan 160°C/Gas 4. Butter a shallow ovenproof dish.

Top and tail the rhubarb, then cut it into 2–3cm lengths and arrange it in the prepared dish. Zest the orange directly over the rhubarb. Sprinkle the sugar over the rhubarb, then juice the orange and drizzle this over too.

For the topping, rub the flour and cinnamon into the butter, then mix in the sugar and oats. Add a pinch of salt. Sprinkle this over the rhubarb, making sure it stays quite loose and not packed down. Dot with some small knobs of butter.

Bake in the oven for about 40 minutes until the rhubarb is tender and the topping is golden brown.

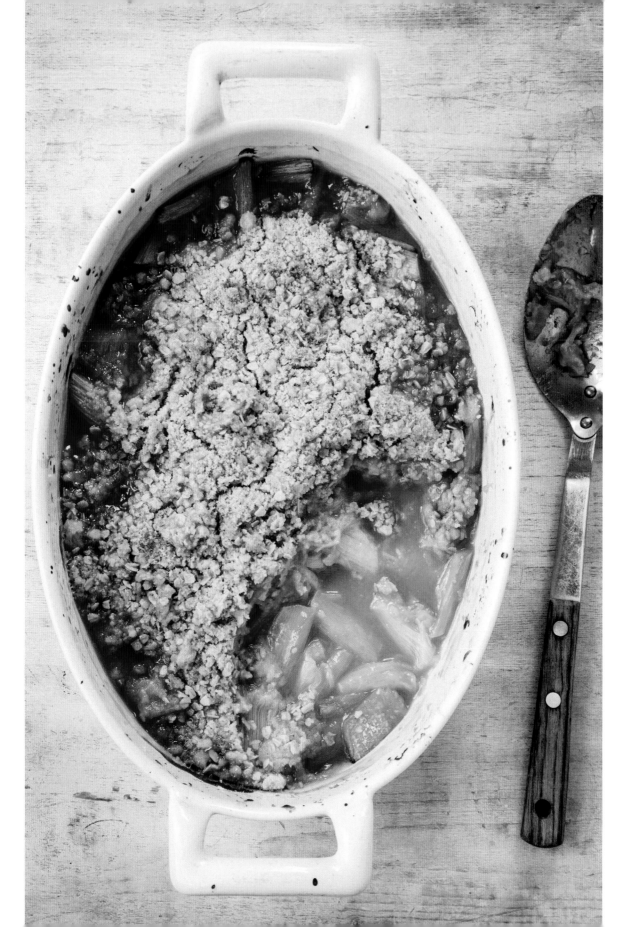

Fruits of the forest cobbler

Cobblers are dead easy to make and for this one we use a bag of frozen fruits of the forest, so there's no prep to do on the fruit. We make no apologies for wanting an easy life. And you can rustle this up at any time of year, even in the depths of winter.

Serves 4

butter, for greasing

300g bag of frozen fruits
    of the forest, defrosted

1 tbsp caster sugar

½ tsp cinnamon

1 tsp cornflour

Topping

150g self-raising flour

½ heaped tsp baking powder

25g caster sugar

pinch of salt

100ml buttermilk

1 few drops of almond extract

1 egg

Preheat the oven to 180°C/Fan 160°C/Gas 4. Butter an ovenproof pan or oven dish, add the defrosted fruit and sprinkle over the sugar and cinnamon. Mix the cornflour with 2 tablespoons of water, then pour this over the fruit and stir well.

For the topping, put the flour, baking powder and sugar in a bowl with a pinch of salt and mix thoroughly. Whisk the buttermilk, almond extract and egg until well combined, then mix with the dry ingredients – the mixture will be soft and sticky, slightly looser than dumplings.

Place heaped tablespoons of the dough over the fruit, then bake in the preheated oven for 30–35 minutes until cooked through. Serve with cream.

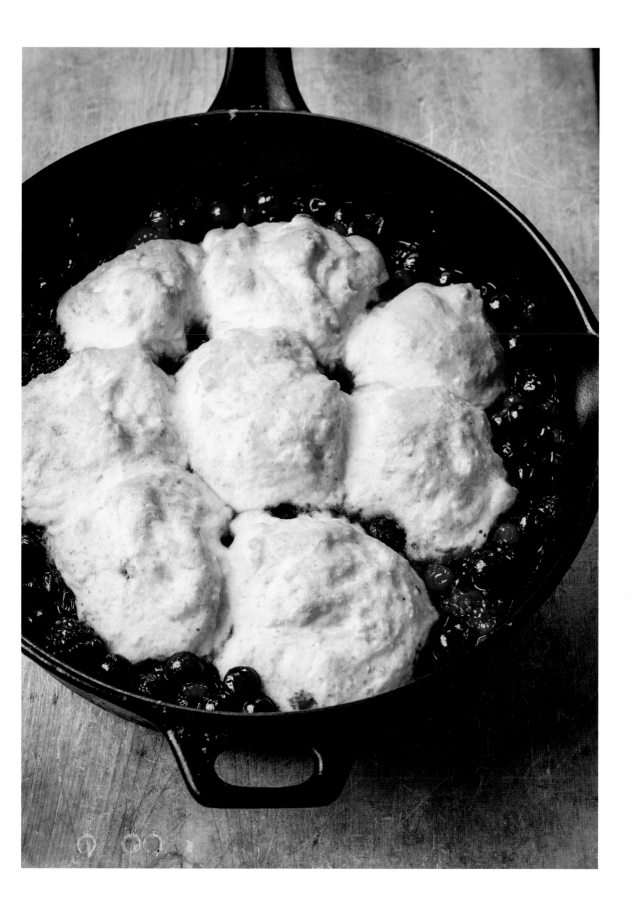

Lemon surprise pudding

This is actually a vegan version of a classic pud and we reckon it's every bit as delicious as the dairy one. The surprise is that the mixture separates into sponge and a delicious runny sauce. Good served with coconut yoghurt if you fancy.

Serves 4

4 tbsp vegetable oil, plus extra for greasing
300g self-raising flour
225g caster sugar
zest of 2 lemons
pinch of salt
250ml coconut milk

Sauce
125g caster sugar
200ml just-boiled water
150ml lemon juice

Preheat the oven to 180°C/Fan 160°C/Gas 4. Lightly oil a large, shallow oven dish.

Mix the flour, sugar and lemon zest together with a pinch of salt. Whisk in the coconut milk and the 4 tablespoons of vegetable oil to make a batter, then spoon this into the prepared dish.

For the sauce, mix the sugar, water and lemon juice together, then pour this over the batter. Bake the pudding in the oven for about 35 minutes, or until the top is springy to touch and golden brown. The sauce will probably be bubbling around the sides.

Remove the dish from the oven and leave the pudding to rest for 10–15 minutes before serving. The sauce will look very runny at first, but it will thicken up as it stands.

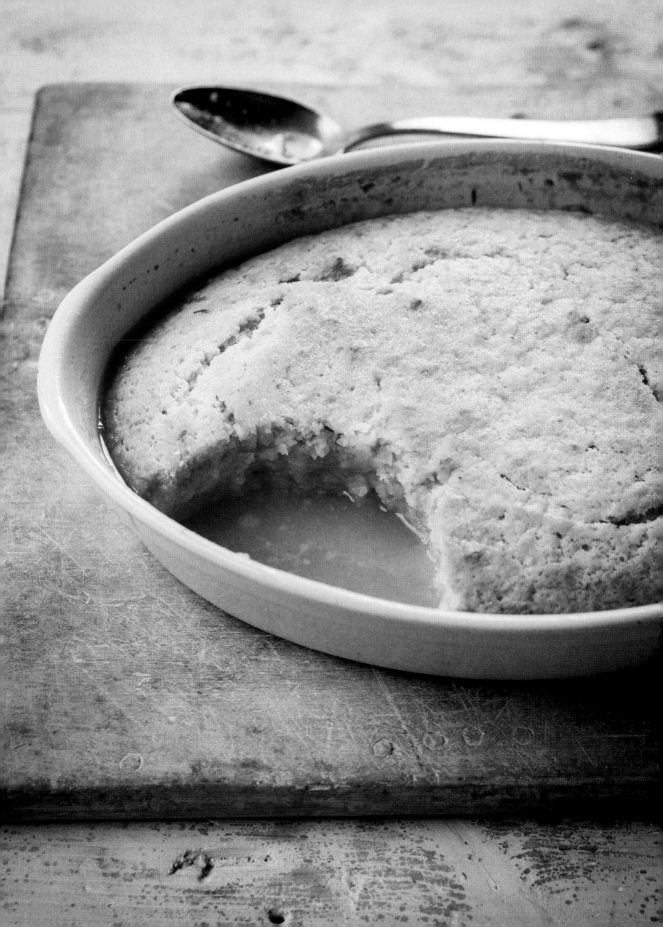

Black Forest pudding

Self-saucing puddings like this are little miracles. You bung everything in the baking dish and it magically separates into moist sponge and gooey sauce. We like to add a drop of the hard stuff, but if you don't fancy it, leave it out and the pud is still fab. The simplest Black Forest gateau you've ever seen.

Serves 4–6

butter, for greasing

400g frozen black cherries, defrosted

Sponge
125g self-raising flour
200g light soft brown sugar
50g cocoa powder
pinch of salt
125ml milk
60ml vegetable oil

Sauce
50g cocoa powder
100g muscovado sugar
150ml just-boiled water
25ml Kirsch or rum (optional)

To serve
double cream

Preheat the oven to 180°C/Fan 160°C/Gas 4. Butter a 2-litre pudding dish, then tip in the cherries – no need to strain them. Give the dish a shake so they are evenly distributed.

For the sponge, mix the self-raising flour with the light soft brown sugar, cocoa powder and a generous pinch of salt. Whisk the milk and vegetable oil together and then pour them over the dry ingredients. Mix until you have a smooth batter, then spoon this over the cherries.

For the sauce, mix the cocoa with the muscovado sugar and sprinkle this evenly over the batter. Pour over the water and Kirsch, if using. Bake the pudding in the oven for 30–35 minutes. The top will turn into a cracked chocolate sponge and the bottom will have a rich, chocolatey sauce around the cherries. If the sponge is still wet in the middle, continue to cook for a few more minutes. If it looks black around the edges, don't worry, it won't be burnt.

Serve hot or at room temperature (the sauce will thicken as it cools) with cream.

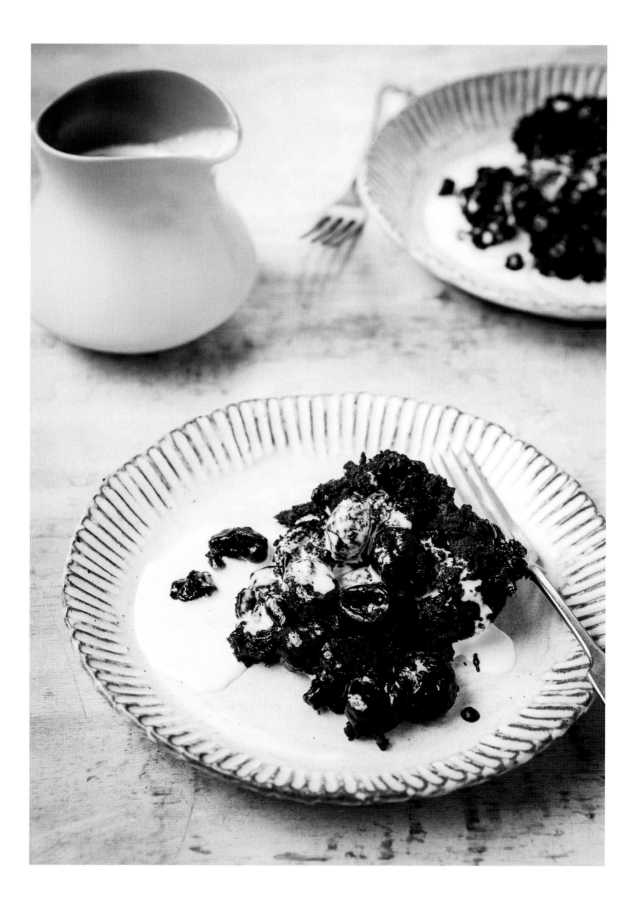

Spiced baked plums

Sometimes a bowlful of simple baked fruit is all you need. These easy but classy baked plums are topped with a lightly spiced, crunchy mixture that melts and caramelises as it cooks – scrumptious! Perfect with some cream or vanilla ice cream.

Serves 4

12 plums, halved and stoned
50g butter, softened
50g soft light brown sugar
½ tsp ground cardamom
pinch of cinnamon
pinch of ground ginger
zest of ½ lemon
½ slice of brioche, panettone or any sponge cake, crumbled

Preheat the oven to 200°C/Fan 180°C/Gas 6. Arrange the plums in a single layer in a baking dish, cut-side up.

Mix the butter with the sugar, spices, zest and crumbled brioche or cake. Divide this mixture between the plums, spooning it into the cavities left by the stones.

Bake the plums in the oven for 15 minutes until they're tender and the topping has lightly caramelised.

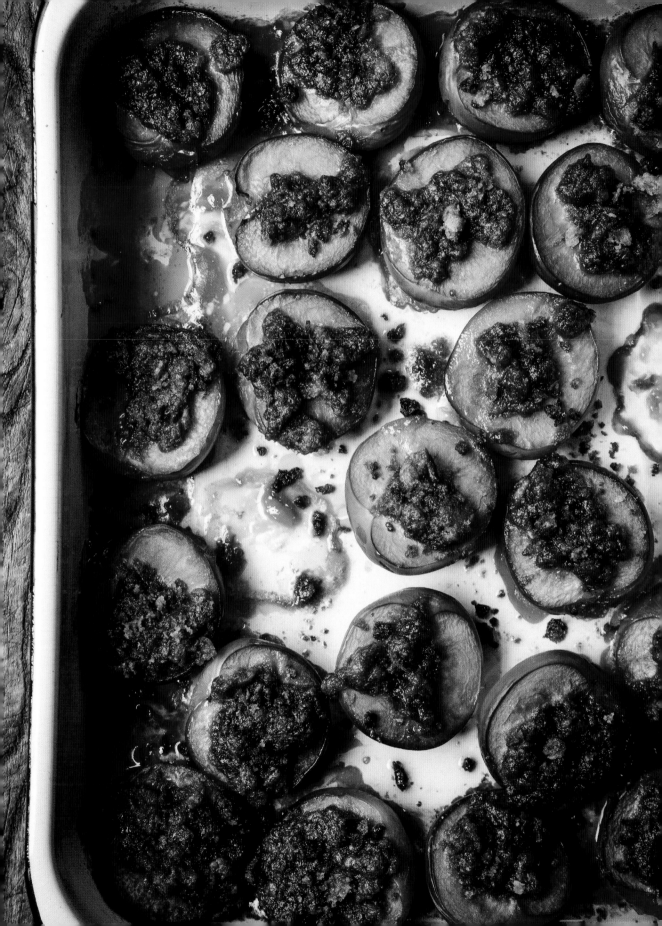

Pear and almond tart

Fruit tarts are so easy to make with ready-rolled puff pastry and we get the all-butter type for the best flavour. We use canned pears and some shop-bought choc sauce for this, so couldn't be quicker and simpler, but if you'd like to make your own sauce, have a look at the recipe on page 276. Impressive and easy.

Serves 4

1 x 320g sheet of ready-rolled puff pastry

1 egg, beaten

a few drops of almond extract (optional)

1 tsp ground cardamom

50g icing sugar

125g ground almonds

400g can of pears in syrup

icing sugar, for dusting

To serve

2 tbsp chocolate sauce (optional)

Preheat the oven to 200°C/Fan 180°C/Gas 6. Unroll the puff pastry sheet on to a baking tray and score a 2cm border all the way around. Brush the pastry with a little of the beaten egg.

Add the almond extract, if using, to the rest of the egg, then mix with the ground cardamom, icing sugar and ground almonds. The mixture should clump together and look a bit like crumble topping. Sprinkle it over the puff pastry, making sure it stays within the scored border.

Drain the pears, reserving the syrup, and slice them thinly. Arrange the slices over the ground almond mixture and dust with icing sugar.

Bake the tart in the oven for about 25 minutes until the pastry has puffed up and turned a rich golden brown and the pears have taken on some colour. Brush the pears and the pastry with some of the pear syrup, then drizzle with the chocolate sauce, if using.

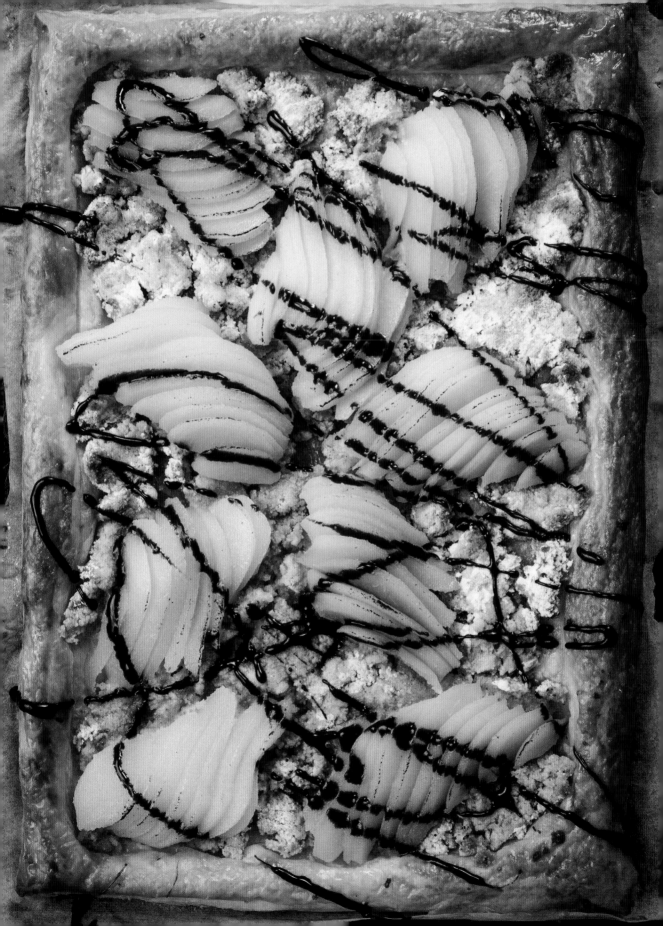

Tropical rice pudding

A tropical take on rice pudding, this has hints of ginger and lime and is finished with coconut cream and pineapple or mango. It makes us think of Caribbean beaches. If you bought a jar of stem ginger for the granola on page 18, this is a great way of using it up.

Serves 4

75g dried pineapple or
    mango, diced
100ml ginger wine
2 tbsp chopped stem ginger
1 strip of pared lime zest
1 tsp mixed spice
3 tbsp light soft brown sugar
pinch of salt
200g pudding rice
1.2 litres milk
100ml coconut cream
100g fresh or tinned pineapple
    or mango (optional)

To serve
ginger wine

Put the dried pineapple or mango and ginger wine in a large saucepan. Bring to the boil and simmer until most of the wine has been absorbed and the dried fruit is plump and softened. Add the chopped stem ginger, lime zest, spice and sugar and stir until the sugar has dissolved, then add a pinch of salt and the rice.

Stir the rice to coat it in the flavourings, then pour in the milk and bring to the boil. Turn the heat down to a simmer and cook, stirring often, until the rice has absorbed much of the milk and has swelled up and softened. This will take 25–30 minutes.

Stir in the coconut cream and the pineapple or mango, if using, to heat through. Serve with a little drizzle of ginger wine.

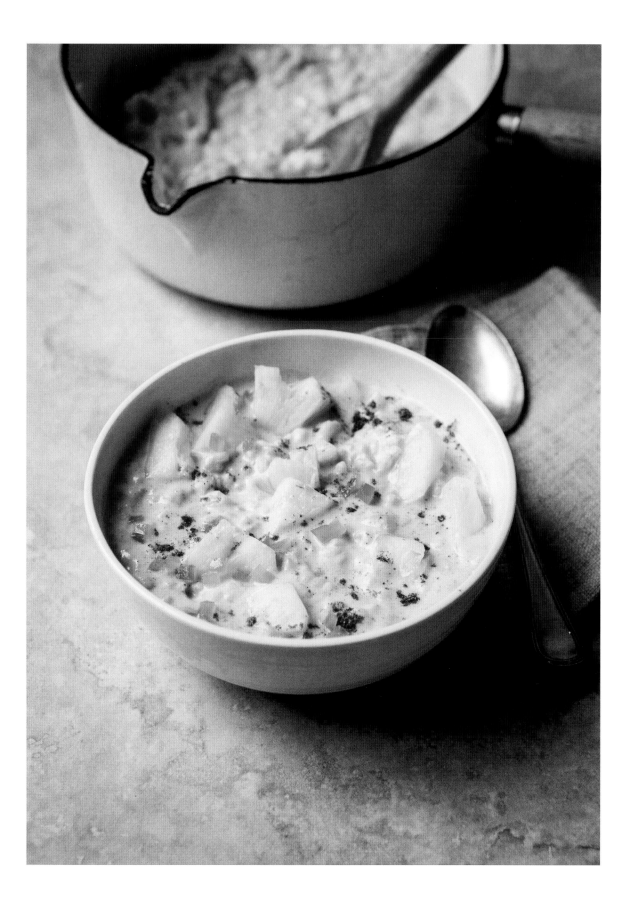

Christmas bread and butter pudding

Bread and butter pud is a real crowd-pleaser and this is our special festive version. Make it with some of that lovely Italian panettone you see around at Christmas and some mincemeat and you might find you prefer it to the trad pud. If you don't have any panettone, brioche also works well. And this is not just for Christmas. If you still have some panettone and mincemeat hanging about by Easter, this is an excellent way of using them up.

Serves 4–6

butter, at room temperature, for spreading, plus extra for greasing

8 slices of panettone

100g mincemeat

2 tbsp whisky (optional)

50g orange curd

4 eggs

50g light soft brown sugar

250ml milk

250ml single cream

1 tbsp demerara sugar

To serve

single cream

Preheat the oven to 180°C/Fan 160°C/Gas 4. Generously butter a 1.5 litre oven dish.

Butter the slices of panettone and cut each slice into 4 triangles. Arrange half of these over the buttered oven dish, buttered-side up. Mix the mincemeat with the whisky, if using, then spoon this over the bread. Add spoonfuls of orange curd, then arrange the remaining slices of panettone on top, buttered-side up again.

Whisk the eggs with the sugar, then add the milk and cream and whisk until smooth. Strain the mixture through a sieve into a jug, then pour it, slowly and steadily, over the pudding. Allow time for it to soak in as you go, so the slices of bread do not float up.

Sprinkle the pudding with the demerara sugar and leave it to stand for 20 minutes. Bake in the oven for 35–40 minutes until the top layer of bread is glossy, crisp and well browned. Serve with cream.

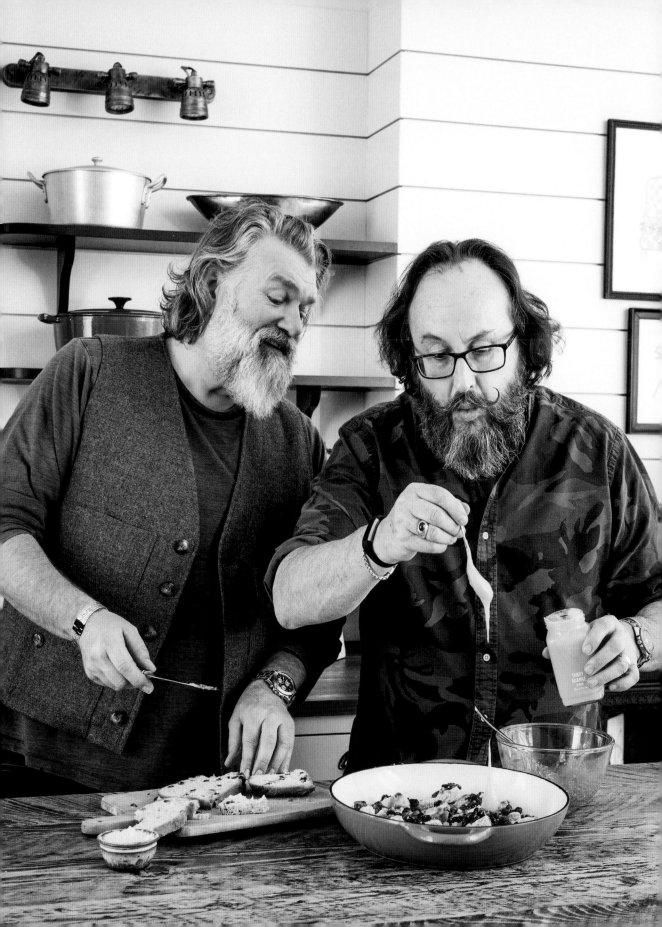

Pimms summer pudding

Pimms and summer pudding both conjure up images of hot sunny afternoons, so put the two together and we're in heaven. This was our invention but when we made it live on Saturday Kitchen, it collapsed, but that was because we didn't line the dish with cling film. Even after national humiliation, we still return to this pudding time and time again. You do have to start the preparation a couple of days ahead, but it's all very easy and this makes a great dish for serving to friends, as you can get it all ready well in advance.

Serves 4–6

200g caster sugar

1 tbsp mint leaves – preferably peppermint or spearmint

250ml Pimms

250g strawberries, hulled and quartered

250g raspberries

250g blueberries

250g redcurrants, taken off their stalks

vegetable oil, for greasing

1 large white sandwich loaf

To serve
fresh berries
clotted or single cream

First, put 50g of the sugar in a spice grinder or food processor with the mint and blitz to a powder. Mix this with the remaining sugar and put it in a pan with the Pimms. Heat gently until the sugar has dissolved, then add all the fruit. Bring up to simmering point and cook for 2 minutes, then strain the fruit through a sieve over a bowl to catch the syrup. Return the syrup to the pan and simmer for 5 minutes until it has thickened slightly. Cool and put the fruit and the syrup in the fridge until the following day.

You need a 2-litre pudding basin. If you are nervous about turning the pudding out, oil the basin lightly and line it with cling film. Cut the bread into 16 slices and remove the crusts. Cut each slice in half. Start assembling the pudding by brushing one side of each slice of bread with syrup and arranging them, syrup-side down, around the base and sides of the pudding basin. Make sure the slices overlap, so no cracks or gaps can appear. This should take about two-thirds of the bread.

Spoon the fruit into the basin, then arrange the remaining bread on top. Cover with a plate small enough to sit just inside the basin, then weight it down – a couple of tins will do the trick. Leave the pudding and the rest of the syrup in the fridge overnight.

When you are ready to serve, turn the pudding out on to a plate and brush with some of the fruit syrup. Garnish with a tumble of extra berries and serve with the remaining syrup and some clotted or single cream.

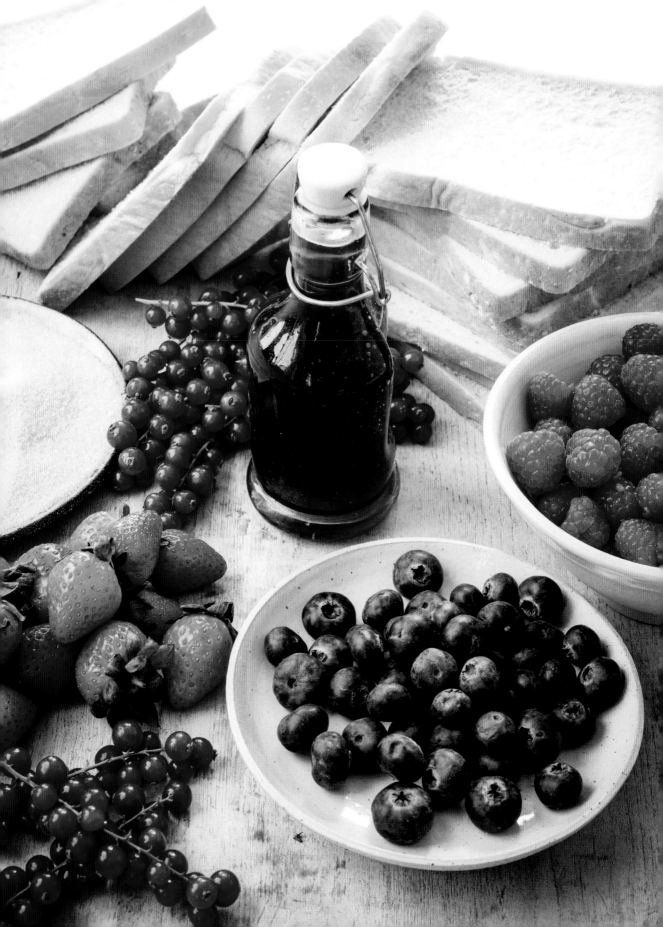

Key lime pie with marshmallows

This is a really simple stripped down version of an American classic, given a genius new look with a topping of toasted marshmallows. Not one for diet days, this, but totally yum.

Serves 6

250g biscuits (gingernut, digestive or chocolate digestive)
100g butter

Filling
300g cream cheese
397g can of condensed milk
zest and juice of 4 limes

Topping
large bag of white marshmallows, halved

Put the biscuits in a bag and crush them with a mallet or rolling pin. Alternatively, put them in a food processor and blitz to fine crumbs. Melt the butter in a small pan and add the biscuit crumbs. Stir to combine, then press into a 23cm loose-bottomed cake tin. Place in the fridge to chill and firm up.

Put the cream cheese in a bowl and beat it with a spoon to soften. Stir in the condensed milk and whisk until smooth – the mixture will look very liquid at this point, but don't worry. Whisk in the lime juice and zest and you will see that the mixture instantly thickens. Pour this on top of the biscuit base and smooth it down, then leave to chill for several hours.

Make sure the filling is well chilled and set. Heat your grill to its highest setting. Arrange the marshmallows over the top of the pie, making sure it is completely covered. Put the pie under the grill very briefly – 20–30 seconds – until the marshmallows are toasted. Alternatively, go over them lightly with a blowtorch if you have one. Run a knife around the edge of the pie, then remove it from the tin. Serve immediately.

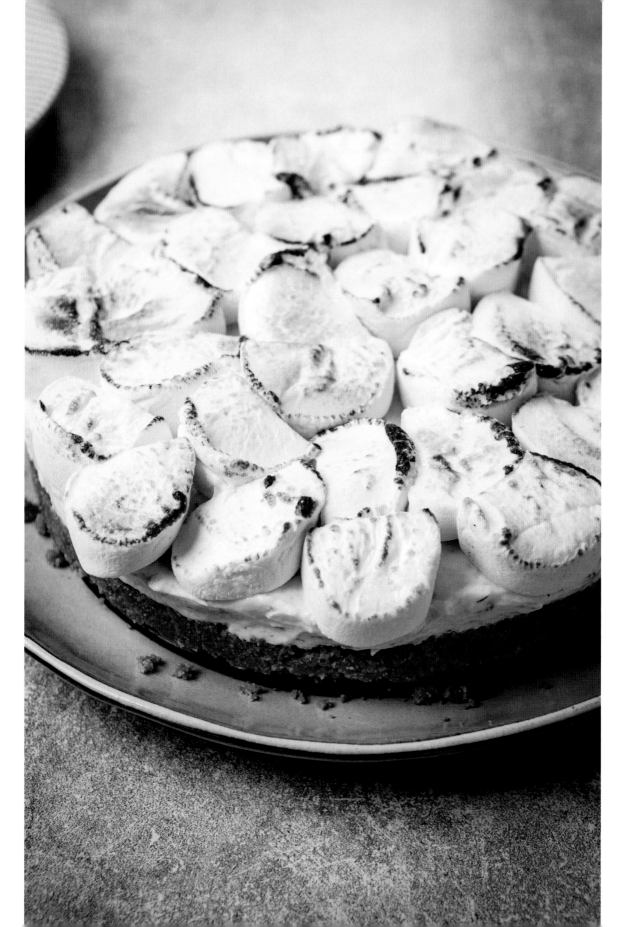

Butterscotch steamed pudding

We both loved steamed puddings when we were kids and we still do. In this one, you line the basin with a paste of sugar and butter and this turns into gooey butterscotch sauce. Need we say more? The sponge is made by the all-in-one method, but make sure the butter is really soft so there are no lumps of butter in the batter. Try saying that last bit quickly!

Serves 6

Sauce
75g butter, softened
75g light soft brown sugar

Sponge
175g butter, very soft
175g light soft brown sugar
175g self-raising flour
3 eggs
1 tbsp milk

To serve
cream or custard

For the sauce, mix the butter and sugar together into a grainy paste. Spread it over the base and sides of a 1.2 litre pudding basin, making sure the thickest layer is on the bottom. Set aside.

Put all the ingredients for the sponge into a food processor or a stand mixer and mix together until you have a batter with a dropping consistency. Be careful not to overwork it.

Pile the batter into the pudding basin and smooth it down. Cover the basin with either a lid or with a pleated layer of foil, secured by string or a couple of elastic bands. Put an upturned heatproof saucer or a folded tea towel in a large, deep pan and put the pudding basin on top. Add enough just-boiled water to come halfway up the sides of the basin. Cover the pan with a tight-fitting lid and place over a low heat, then leave the pudding to steam in the gently simmering water for about 2½ hours. Keep an eye on the water level and add more boiling water when necessary. Check for doneness by inserting a skewer into the centre of the pudding – it should come out clean.

Remove the pudding from the steamer and run a palette knife around the edge, just to make sure it is loose enough to turn out. Cover with a plate and turn upside down, then lever off the basin – take care, the basin will be hot. The butter and sugar should have melted together into a sauce around the steamed sponge. Serve with cream or custard.

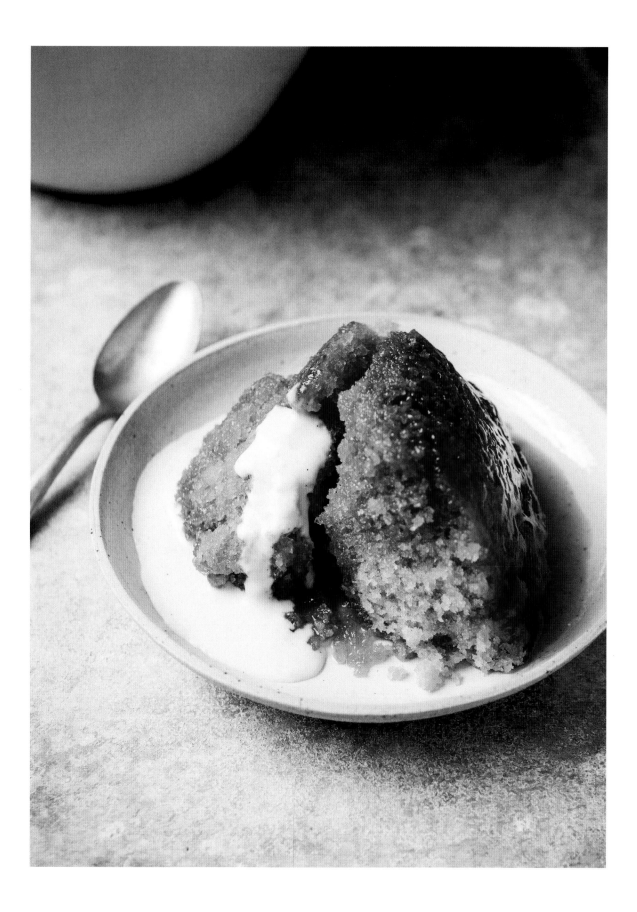

Irish coffee ice cream

This ice cream doesn't need churning so is incredibly easy to make – just mix and shove it in the freezer. The condensed milk and the whiskey stop it from going rock solid as it freezes. A treat for the grown-ups and what a way to finish off your dinner. We've been known to enjoy a glass of Irish whiskey on the side.

Serves 6

4 tbsp instant espresso powder

50ml just-boiled water

600ml double cream

397g can of condensed milk

1 tsp vanilla extract

3 tbsp Irish whiskey

100g chocolate-coated coffee beans

Dissolve the instant espresso powder in the water and set aside. Using an electric hand whisk, beat the double cream until it starts to thicken and aerate. Gradually add the condensed milk, followed by the vanilla extract, espresso mixture and Irish whiskey. Keep whisking until you get a uniform colour and consistency.

Stir in the coffee beans, then transfer the mixture to a freezer-proof container. Freeze for several hours until solid, then serve straight from the freezer.

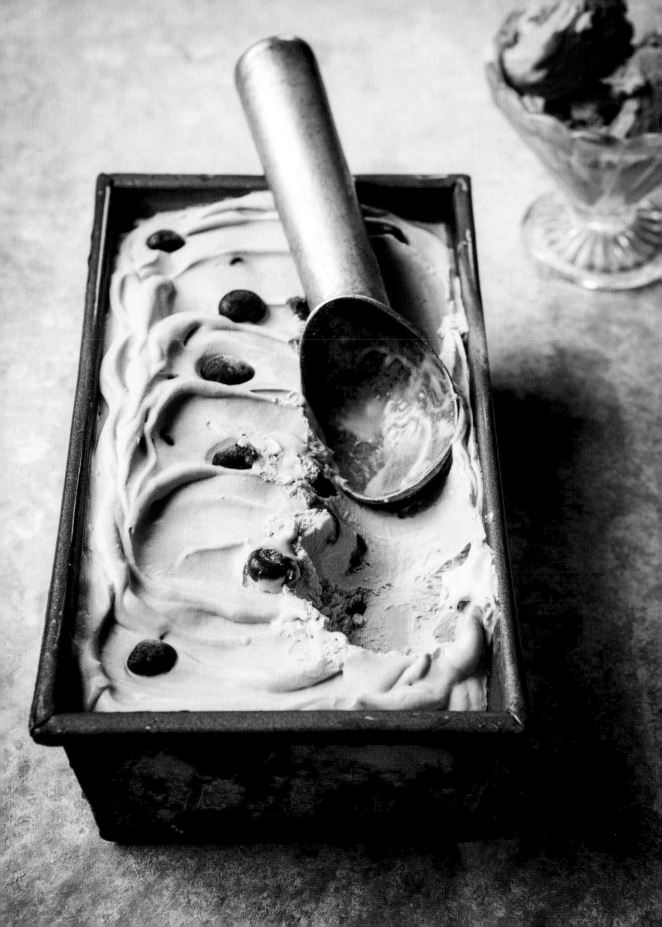

Boozy syllabub trifle

Everyone loves a trifle. This pudding looks very posh but it's really just an assembly job. You have to mix the syllabub, but the rest of the work is just piling things into a bowl. Not too hard really when you think of the treat you have in store. Shop-bought custard is fine or make your own with the recipe on page 277.

Serves 6

1 packet of trifle sponges or
    fingers
2–3 tbsp raspberry jam
100ml sweet sherry or marsala
150g amaretti biscuits
500g raspberries
1 large pot of custard
50g toasted flaked almonds

Syllabub

50ml sweet sherry or marsala
1 tbsp brandy (optional)
zest of 1 lemon, plus extra
    to garnish
2 tbsp caster sugar
400ml whipping cream

First start the syllabub. Put the sweet sherry or marsala in a bowl with the brandy, if using, the lemon zest and caster sugar. Stir until the sugar has dissolved. Leave this to stand for at least the time it takes to assemble the trifle, but for several hours if you are able to prepare ahead.

To assemble the trifle, first spread half the trifle sponges or fingers with the raspberry jam and arrange them in the base of a trifle bowl. Pour over the sherry and top with the amaretti biscuits, followed by the raspberries. Spoon the custard over the raspberries, then cover and leave to chill.

Now finish the syllabub. Whip the cream until it reaches the soft peak stage, then stir in the sherry mixture and whisk again to combine. Spoon this over the trifle, then sprinkle over the toasted almonds and some extra lemon zest.

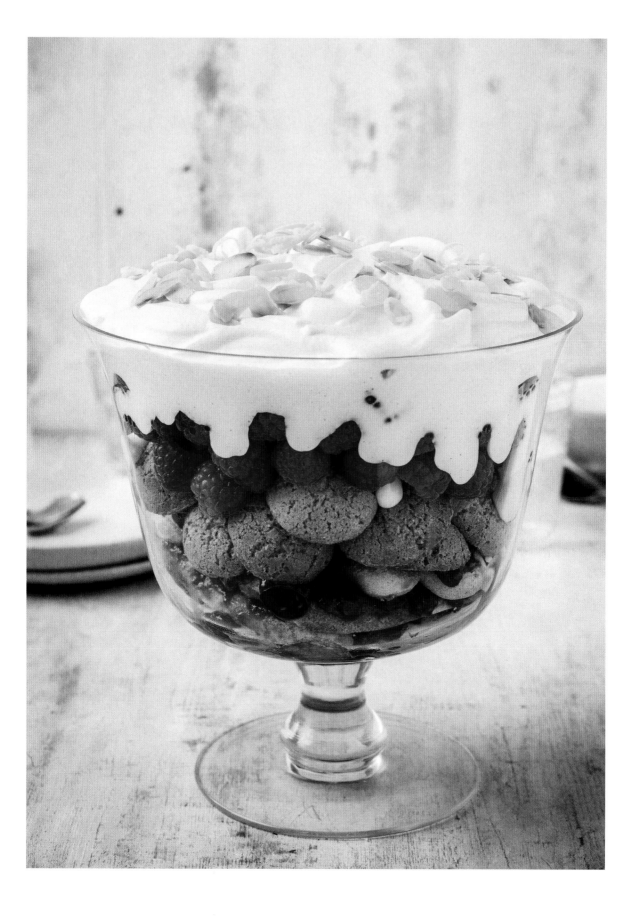

Upside-down blueberry tray bake

A cross between a tray bake and an upside-down cake, this is great for teatime or for pudding with cream. It's good to look at and great to eat.

Makes 12 slices

Blueberry layer

25g butter, softened, plus extra
    for greasing
50g caster sugar
500g blueberries

Cake

300g butter, softened
200g caster sugar
50g honey
1 tsp vanilla extract
225g self-raising flour
75g fine cornmeal
1 tsp baking powder
4 eggs
1 tbsp milk

Grease a 20 x 30cm baking tin with butter and line it with baking paper. If the tin has a loose bottom or side, wrap it in a single layer of foil to stop any blueberry juice leaking out.

Smear the 25g of butter over the base of the lined tin, then sprinkle with the sugar. Arrange the blueberries over the base of the tin – if the blueberries are large and fat, there should be just enough to cover the butter and sugar in a single layer.

Put all the ingredients for the cake into a large bowl and beat together with an electric hand whisk. Take care not to over mix. If the butter is a little on the firm side, beat this first before adding everything else. Alternatively, put everything in a food processor. Add a little more milk, if necessary to get a dropping consistency, then spoon the mixture over the blueberries. Make sure they are completely covered and smooth the top down.

Bake in the oven for 30–35 minutes until the cake has slightly shrunk away from the sides and is springy to touch. A skewer inserted into the centre should come out clean.

If you want to serve this warm as a dessert with cream, turn it out immediately or cut slices directly from the tin. If you prefer to serve it as a cake, leave to cool in the tin, then upturn on to a board and cut into squares.

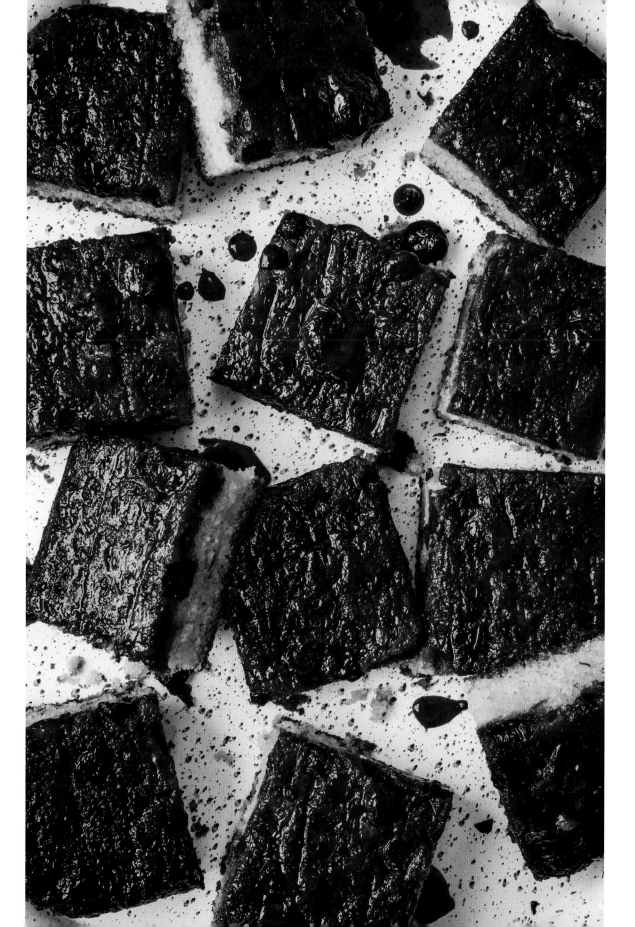

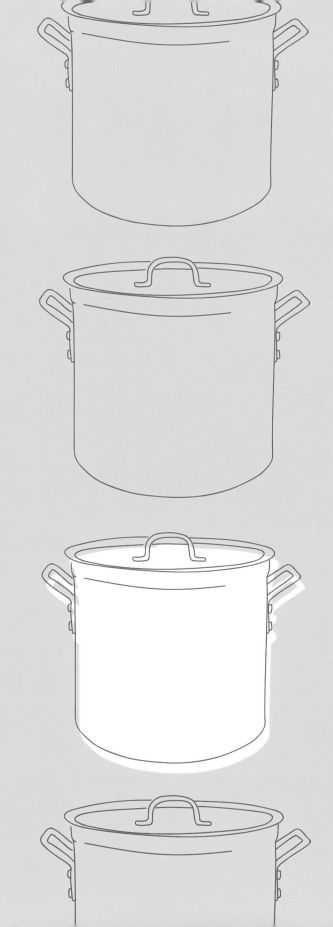

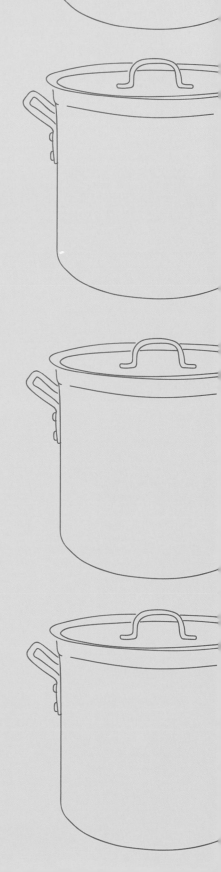

Basics

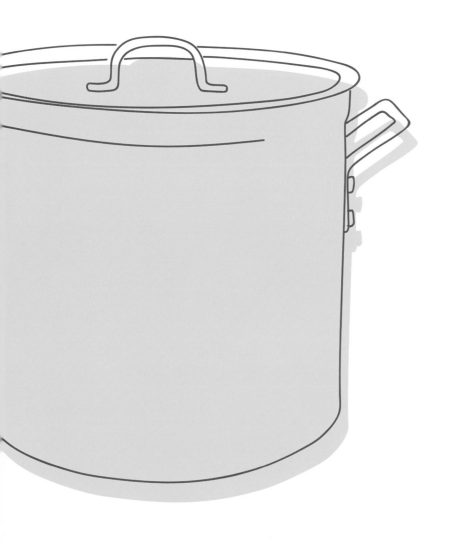

Vegetable stock

This is a good basic vegetable stock for soups and veggie dishes.

Makes about 1.5 litres

---

1 tsp olive oil

2 large onions, roughly chopped

3 large carrots, chopped

200g squash or pumpkin, unpeeled and diced

4 celery sticks, sliced

2 leeks, sliced

100ml white wine or vermouth

large thyme sprig

large parsley sprig

1 bay leaf

a few peppercorns

Heat the olive oil in a large pan. Add all the vegetables and fry them over a high heat, stirring regularly, until they start to brown and caramelise around the edges. This will take at least 10 minutes. Add the white wine or vermouth and boil until it has evaporated away.

Cover the veg with 2 litres of water and add the herbs and peppercorns. Bring to the boil, then turn the heat down to a gentle simmer. Cook the stock, uncovered, for about an hour, stirring every so often.

Check the stock – the colour should have some depth to it. Strain it through a colander or a sieve lined with muslin or kitchen paper into a bowl and store it in the fridge for up to a week. Alternatively, pour the stock into freezer-proof containers and freeze.

Spring vegetable stock

A lovely fresh-tasting stock to make if you have asparagus trimmings and fresh pea pods.

Makes about 1.5 litres

2 large onions, roughly chopped,

3 large carrots, well washed, chopped

1 fennel bulb, roughly chopped

4 celery sticks, sliced

2 leeks, sliced

pea pods

asparagus trimmings

100ml white wine or vermouth

large tarragon sprig

large parsley sprig

1 bay leaf

a few peppercorns

Put all the vegetables in a large saucepan, add the white wine or vermouth and boil until the alcohol has evaporated away.

Cover the vegetables with 2 litres of water and add the herbs and peppercorns. Bring the water to the boil, then turn the heat down to a gentle simmer. Cook the stock, uncovered, for 20 minutes, stirring every so often. It's nice to keep the fresh green colour so don't cook it for longer.

Strain the stock through a colander or a sieve lined with muslin or kitchen paper into a bowl and store in the fridge for up to a week. Alternatively, pour the stock into freezer-proof containers and freeze.

Fish stock

You can buy fish stock but if it's nice to make your own when you have time and stash it in the freezer. Fishmongers are always happy to provide fish heads and bones.

Makes about 1.5 litres

2kg fish heads and bones from white fish (ask your fishmonger)

1 tbsp salt

2 tbsp olive oil

1 onion, finely chopped

2 leeks, finely sliced

½ fennel bulb, finely chopped

1 celery stick, sliced

2 garlic cloves, sliced

200ml white wine

bouquet garni (2 sprigs each of parsley, tarragon and thyme)

2 bay leaves

a few peppercorns

1 piece of thinly pared lemon zest

Put the fish heads and bones in a bowl, cover them with cold water and add the salt. Leave them to stand for an hour, then drain and wash thoroughly under running water. This process helps to draw out any blood from the fish and gives you a much clearer, fresher-tasting stock.

Heat the olive oil in a large saucepan. Add the onion, leeks, fennel, celery and garlic. Cook the vegetables over a medium heat for several minutes until they have started to soften without taking on any colour.

Add the fish heads and bones and pour over the wine. Bring to the boil, then add 2 litres of water. Bring back to the boil, skim off any mushroom-coloured foam that appears, then turn the heat down to a very slow simmer. Add the herbs, peppercorns and lemon zest and leave to simmer for half an hour, skimming off any foam every so often.

Strain the stock through a colander or sieve, then line the sieve with muslin or kitchen paper and strain the stock again – do not push it through as that will result in a cloudier stock. Transfer the stock to a container and chill it in the fridge. You can keep the stock in the fridge for 3–4 days or freeze it.

Chicken stock

You can make a decent chicken stock from one carcass but it's even better with two or three, so freeze your carcasses until you have a few. And if you add a few chicken wings it tastes even better.

Makes about 1 litre

at least 1 chicken carcass, pulled apart

4 chicken wings (optional)

1 onion, left unpeeled, cut into quarters

1 large carrot, cut into large chunks

2 celery sticks, roughly chopped

1 leek, roughly chopped

1 tsp black peppercorns

3 bay leaves

large thyme sprig

large parsley sprig

a few garlic cloves, unpeeled (optional)

Put the chicken bones and the wings, if using, into a pan. It should be just large enough for the carcass or carcasses to be quite a snug fit. Cover with cold water, bring to the boil, then skim off any foam that collects. Add all the remaining ingredients and turn the heat down to a very low simmer. Partially cover the pan with a lid.

Leave the stock to simmer for about 3 hours, then remove the pan from the heat. Line a sieve or colander with muslin or kitchen paper and place a bowl underneath the sieve, then ladle the stock through to strain it. Decant the stock into a container and leave to cool.

The stock can be used immediately, although it is best to skim off most of the fat that will collect on the top. If you don't need the stock immediately, chill it in the fridge. The fat will set on top (and can be used for frying) and will be much easier to remove. You can keep the stock in the fridge for up to 5 days or freeze it.

Beef stock

This tasty stock is a good basis for any meat soup or casserole. Your butcher will be happy to give you bones and you could ask for some beef trimmings as well, or get yourself a piece of beef shin.

Makes about 2 litres

1.5 kg beef bones, including marrow bones if possible, cut into small lengths

500g beef trimmings or beef shin

2 onions, unpeeled and roughly chopped

1 leek, roughly chopped

2 celery sticks, roughly chopped

2 carrots, roughly chopped

2 tomatoes

$\frac{1}{2}$ tsp peppercorns

a bouquet garni (large thyme sprigs, parsley and 2 bay leaves)

Put the bones and meat into a large stockpot and cover them with cold water – at least 3–3.5 litres. Bring the water to the boil and when a starchy, mushroom-grey foam appears, start skimming. Keep on skimming as the foam turns white and continue until it has almost stopped developing.

Add the vegetables, peppercorns and bouquet garni, turn down the heat until the stock is simmering very gently, then partially cover the pan with a lid. Leave the stock to simmer for 3–4 hours.

Line a sieve or colander with 2 layers of muslin or a tea towel and place it over a large bowl or saucepan. Ladle the stock into the sieve or colander to strain it. Remove the meat and set it aside, then discard everything else.

Pour the strained stock into large container and chill it thoroughly. The fat should solidify on top of the stock and will be very easy to remove. Keep the stock in the fridge for 2 or 3 days or freeze it.

Tomato sauce

There are plenty of ready-made tomato sauces in the supermarket but it is cheaper – and better – to make your own when you have time. Make a big batch and freeze it in portions.

Makes about 1 litre

6 tbsp olive oil

2 onions, very finely sliced

6 garlic cloves, finely chopped

250ml red wine

4 x 400g cans of tomatoes or 1.5kg plum tomatoes, peeled and chopped

2 tsp dried oregano

1 tsp fresh thyme leaves

2 bay leaves

pinch of sugar (optional)

salt and black pepper

Heat the olive oil in a large saucepan and add the onions. Sauté them very gently until soft – this will take at least 15 minutes.

Add the garlic and cook for another 3–4 minutes over a very gentle heat, then pour in the red wine. Boil until the wine is reduced by at least half, then add the tomatoes and herbs. Season with salt and pepper.

Bring the sauce to the boil, then turn down the heat, cover the pan and simmer for an hour. At this point taste the sauce and if it seems too acidic, add a generous pinch of sugar. Continue to simmer, uncovered, for about 30 minutes until well reduced. Use immediately or leave to cool and then store in the fridge or freeze.

Mild curry powder

A mild, sweet mixture that works well for the keema peas recipe (see page 168) and would also be good in a creamy chicken curry. There's just a hint of chilli, which makes this a good curry powder to use when cooking for young children.

Makes 1 small jar

1 tbsp coriander seeds

1 tsp cumin seeds

1 tsp fennel seeds

½ tsp aniseed (optional)

½ tsp fenugreek seeds

¼ tsp white peppercorns

seeds from 6 cardamom pods

4 cloves

4cm piece of cinnamon stick, broken up

2 bay leaves

1 tbsp ground turmeric

¼ tsp cayenne

Put the whole spices and bay leaves into a dry frying pan – preferably not a non-stick one. Toast over a medium heat until the aroma is strong.

Remove from the heat and transfer to a bowl to cool down. Grind to a powder in a spice grinder or with a pestle and mortar, then mix with the turmeric and cayenne. Store in an airtight jar.

Medium curry powder

This spice mix is ideal for the aloo gobi on page 92 and the compliments the other spices included. You can use any strength of chilli powder, depending on how hot you want the mixture.

Makes 1 small jar

1 tbsp cumin seeds

1 tbsp coriander seeds

1 tsp mustard seeds

1 tsp nigella seeds

½ tsp fenugreek seeds

3cm piece of cinnamon stick, broken up

6 dried curry leaves (optional)

1 tsp ground turmeric

1 tsp chilli powder

1 tsp sweet paprika

1 tsp garlic granules

¼ tsp asafoetida

Put all the whole spices and curry leaves into a dry frying pan – preferably not a non-stick one. Toast over a medium heat until the aroma is strong and the mustard seeds are popping.

Transfer the toasted spices and curry leaves to a bowl to cool, then grind to a fine powder in a spice grinder or with a pestle and mortar. Mix with the turmeric, chilli powder, sweet paprika, garlic granules and asafoetida and store in an airtight jar.

West Indian curry powder

A lovely mix for the West Indian curry on page 84 or other Caribbean dishes.

Makes 1 small jar

4 cm piece of cinnamon stick, broken up

2 tbsp coriander seeds

2 tsp cumin seeds

1 tsp mustard seeds

1 tsp white peppercorns

½ tsp allspice berries

½ tsp fenugreek

seeds from 6 cardamom pods

4 cloves

2 mace blades

2 dried bay leaves

1 tbsp ground turmeric

½ tsp onion salt

Put all the whole spices and the bay leaves into a dry frying pan – preferably not a non-stick one. Toast the spices over a medium heat, shaking regularly, until their aroma intensifies and the mustard seeds start popping. Transfer to a bowl and allow to cool.

Grind the spices in a spice grinder or with a pestle and mortar to form a fine powder, then mix with the turmeric and onion salt. Store in an airtight jar.

Laksa paste

Here's a simple recipe if you want to make your own paste for the quick prawn laksa on page 76.

Makes 1 small jar

3 lemongrass stalks, soft white inner parts only, chopped

2 red chillies, deseeded and chopped

4 garlic cloves, roughly chopped

15g fresh root ginger, chopped

1 piece of pared lime zest

2 shallots

1 tbsp shrimp paste

1 tsp light soft brown sugar

1 tsp turmeric

¼ tsp cinnamon

juice of 1 lime

salt and black pepper

Put all the ingredients in a small food processor with plenty of salt and pepper and a splash of water. Process until everything is well broken down and combined. The paste won't be completely smooth but that's fine. Store in the fridge until needed.

Red harissa paste

The long red peppers we use here are traditional, but they aren't particularly hot when deseeded. If you want a bit more heat, use hotter smaller red chillies.

Makes 1 jar

2 red peppers, cut in half
 and deseeded
8 long red chilli peppers,
  halved and deseeded
4 garlic cloves, left unpeeled
1 tsp sea salt
1 tsp cumin seeds
$\frac{1}{2}$ tsp coriander seeds
$\frac{1}{2}$ tsp caraway seeds
1cm piece of cinnamon stick
1 tsp sweet smoked paprika
2 tsp red wine vinegar
2 tbsp olive oil, plus extra for
  storing
salt and black pepper

Preheat the oven to 220°C/Fan 200°C/Gas 7. Put the peppers, chillies and garlic cloves in a roasting tin and roast for 20–25 minutes until the skins have blistered slightly and blackened. Cover the roasting tin with a couple of tea towels or a sheet of foil and leave everything to steam until cool enough to handle. Peel off as much of the skin as you can from the red peppers and the chillies – a little skin is good for texture and charred flavour. Squeeze the garlic flesh out of the skins.

Transfer to a food processor with the sea salt and whizz to form a purée.

Toast the whole spices lightly in a dry frying pan until the aroma is strong, then transfer them to a bowl to cool. Grind the spices in a spice mill or use a pestle and mortar, then add them to the peppers in the food processor. Add the paprika, vinegar and oil, give the mixture another quick blitz, then taste. Add more salt, pepper and vinegar if necessary.

Decant the paste into a jar and drizzle over a little more olive oil to help preserve it. Store in the fridge.

Basil pesto

Pine nuts are traditional in pesto but they are expensive these days and we think almonds work just as well. We like to add a little lemon zest too.

Makes about 250ml

50g pine nuts or blanched almonds

generous pinch of salt

1 garlic clove

leaves from 2 large bunches of basil

zest of ½ lemon

25g Parmesan cheese, grated

up to 150ml extra virgin olive oil, plus extra for storing

Put the pine nuts or almonds in a dry frying pan and toast them, shaking the pan regularly, until they start to turn light brown. Watch them like a hawk as they can burn very quickly. Immediately transfer them to a food processor and leave to cool.

Add the salt and garlic to the processor, then pulse a few times to break up the nuts and garlic. Add the basil and lemon zest and pulse a few more times, pushing the basil down as necessary, to make quite a coarse paste.

Add the Parmesan and start drizzling in the olive oil while continuing to pulse – you want the pesto to be lightly emulsified, but not smooth. Add just enough of the oil to create quite a thick paste. It shouldn't be runny.

Transfer to a jar and top with olive oil to keep the surface fresh. Store in the fridge and use as required.

Red pesto

This pesto is fine without the Parmesan if you would like a vegan sauce.

Makes about 200ml

50g pine nuts

generous pinch of salt

1 garlic clove, roughly
chopped

leaves from a small bunch
of parsley

leaves from a small bunch
of basil

leaves from a sprig of oregano

1 pack of sunblush or
sun-drenched tomatoes
(about 190g)

1 tsp red wine vinegar

50g Parmesan cheese,
grated (optional)

50ml olive oil, plus extra
for storing

Toast the pine nuts in a dry frying pan until lightly golden, then transfer them to a food processor. Add the salt and garlic, then pulse until quite finely chopped. Add the herbs, tomatoes and red wine vinegar and continue to pulse, pushing down the leaves as necessary, until everything is well broken down.

Add the cheese, if using, then with the motor running, drizzle in the olive oil until you have a deep red, green-flecked paste. Transfer the pesto to a jar and cover with a little more olive oil to preserve, then store in the fridge until needed.

Shortcrust pastry

This is a basic shortcrust pastry, suitable for the showstopper quiche on page 128.

Makes about 400g

250g plain flour, plus extra for dusting

150g cold butter, cut into cubes

1 large egg, beaten

Put the flour and butter in a food processor and pulse until the mixture resembles breadcrumbs, or rub the butter into the flour with your fingertips. Add the beaten egg and mix until the mixture is just beginning to come together, then shape the dough into a ball.

Basmati rice

We like to soak our rice for best results, but if you don't have time, rinse it well and cook for 15 minutes, instead of 10.

Serves 4

200g basmati or long-grain rice
generous pinch of salt

Rinse the rice thoroughly until the water runs clear, then put it in a bowl and cover with cold water. Leave to stand for 30 minutes then drain thoroughly and transfer to a pan.

Add a generous pinch of salt and cover with 300ml of water. Bring to the boil, then turn down the heat and leave the rice to cook for 10 minutes. At this point, most of the water should have been absorbed and the rice should have turned from a greyish semi-translucence to an opaque white. Take the pan off the heat.

Fold a tea towel and put it over the pan, then put the lid back on top. Leave the rice to steam for a further 5 minutes – the tea towel will help the rice become fluffy by absorbing excess moisture. Fluff the rice up with a fork and serve.

How to cook chickpeas

Chickpeas take longer to cook than any other beans/pulses, so this method can be adapted for other beans, but with reduced timings. It is impossible to give really accurate timings because chickpeas vary enormously in size and age – the older they are, the longer they will take. We suggest cooking 500g at a time – more than usually needed for one meal, but it's good to do more, as they take so long to cook and they freeze really well.

500g chickpeas
1 tsp salt

Cover the chickpeas in plenty of cold water then leave them to soak for at least 8 hours, preferably overnight. If you want to speed this up a bit, you can do a 'quick' soak. Put the chickpeas in a pan, cover them with water and bring to the boil for 1 minute. Remove the pan from the heat and leave to stand for an hour.

Drain the chickpeas (regardless of how long you have soaked them) and cover with fresh water. Make sure they have at least 5cm of water over them. Bring to the boil and boil fiercely for 5 minutes, then add a teaspoon of salt and turn the temperature down to a gentle simmer. Cook for at least 45 minutes, stirring gently from time to time just to move them around. Check to see if they are cooked – they can take longer, anything up to an hour and a half, depending on age. If they aren't quite cooked, continue to check every 10–15 minutes.

When the chickpeas are cooked, drain, leave to cool and then store in the fridge or freezer. You can use the cooking liquid as stock for soup.

Chocolate sauce

If you want to make your own choc sauce for the pear tart on page 238, try this. It's excellent poured over ice cream too. Pear eau de vie or an almond liqueur is good, but brandy is fine.

Serves 4

200ml double cream

25g butter, diced

125g dark chocolate (at least 70% cocoa solids), broken up

generous pinch of sea salt

1 tbsp brandy or liqueur (optional)

Put the cream, butter and chocolate into a pan. Add the salt and heat gently until everything has melted. Remove the pan from the heat and whisk until you have a smooth sauce. Add the alcohol, if using, then pour into a jug.

Use the sauce immediately or allow it to cool and transfer to the fridge. The sauce will set to a spreadable consistency and can be used as a spread. To reheat, warm it very gently in a saucepan until it melts, making sure it doesn't boil and separate.

Custard

We've made this quite a thick custard for the trifle on page 252, but if you would like a thinner pouring custard for serving with crumble and puddings, just leave out the cornflour.

Serves 4

300ml whole milk
300ml double cream
1 vanilla pod, split
pinch of salt
4 egg yolks
50g caster sugar
2 tbsp cornflour (optional)

Put the milk and cream into a pan with the vanilla pod and a pinch of salt. Slowly heat until the mixture is almost at boiling point, then remove from the heat and leave to infuse with the vanilla pod until tepid.

Whisk the egg yolks, sugar and cornflour, if using, with electric beaters until pale and mousse-like, then gradually stir in the milk and cream.

Strain the mixture back into the pan, discarding the vanilla pod. Cook over a very low heat, stirring constantly and making sure it doesn't boil, until the mixture thickens. If using cornflour, it may suddenly go from very liquid to thick – whisk thoroughly at this point to make sure no lumps form. If not using cornflour, stir until you can coat the back of a wooden spoon.

Use the custard immediately or transfer it to a jug or bowl and cover with cling film. Make sure the cling film is touching the top of the custard so a skin doesn't form. If you want to reheat the custard, warm it gently in a saucepan and make sure it doesn't boil.

Index

O

P

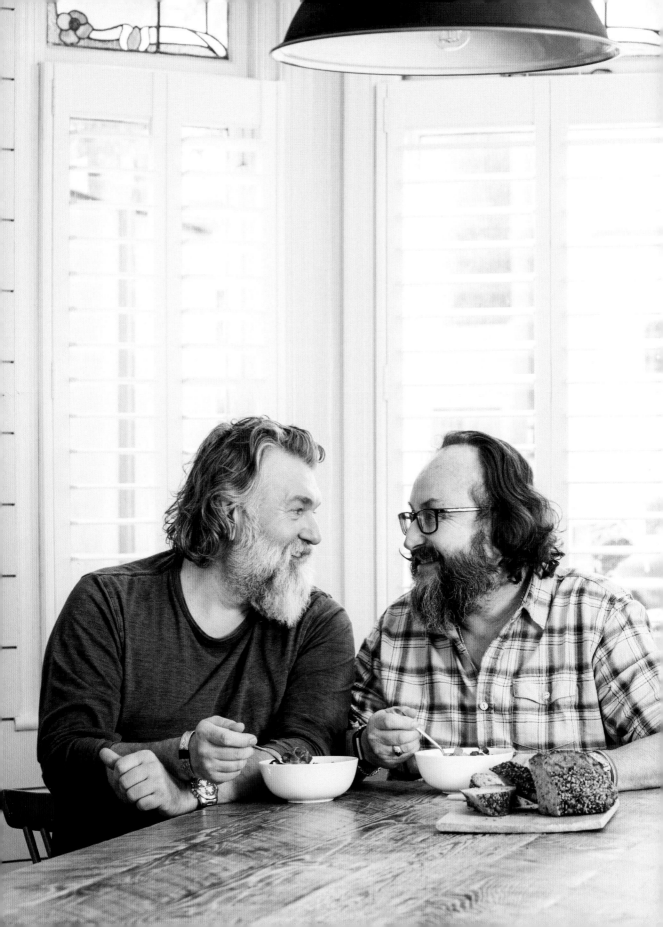

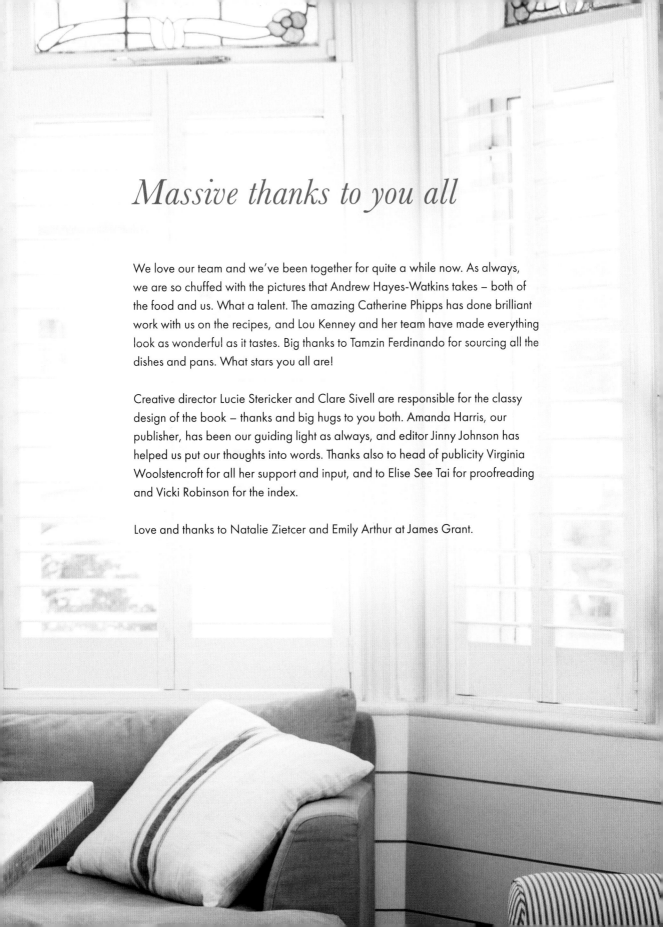

Massive thanks to you all

We love our team and we've been together for quite a while now. As always, we are so chuffed with the pictures that Andrew Hayes-Watkins takes – both of the food and us. What a talent. The amazing Catherine Phipps has done brilliant work with us on the recipes, and Lou Kenney and her team have made everything look as wonderful as it tastes. Big thanks to Tamzin Ferdinando for sourcing all the dishes and pans. What stars you all are!

Creative director Lucie Stericker and Clare Sivell are responsible for the classy design of the book – thanks and big hugs to you both. Amanda Harris, our publisher, has been our guiding light as always, and editor Jinny Johnson has helped us put our thoughts into words. Thanks also to head of publicity Virginia Woolstencroft for all her support and input, and to Elise See Tai for proofreading and Vicki Robinson for the index.

Love and thanks to Natalie Zietcer and Emily Arthur at James Grant.

We'd like to dedicate this book to Lucie Stericker, who's been with us from the start of our wonderful publishing adventure. We make beautiful cookbooks, which is largely down to you, and this one is a supermodel. Love and appreciation, Si and Dave.

First published in Great Britain in 2019 by Seven Dials
an imprint of The Orion Publishing Group Ltd
Carmelite House, 50 Victoria Embankment, London EC4Y 0DZ
An Hachette UK Company

1 3 5 7 9 10 8 6 4 2

A CIP catalogue record for this book is
available from the British Library.

ISBN: 978-1-4091-7193-5
eISBN: 978-1-4091-7194-2

Recipe consultant: Catherine Phipps
Photographer: Andrew Hayes-Watkins
Design and art direction: Lucie Stericker and Clare Sivell
Editor: Jinny Johnson
Food stylist: Lou Kenney
Food stylist's assistants: Evie Harbury, Lara Luck and Sophie Hammond
Prop stylist: Tamzin Ferdinando
Proofreader: Elise See Tai
Indexer: Vicki Robinson
Production manager: Katie Horrocks

Printed and bound in Germany

www.orionbooks.co.uk

For more delicious recipes plus exclusive competitions and sneak
previews from Orion's cookery writers visit kitchentales.co.uk